Common Operations on the Foot

General Editor, Wolfe Surgical Atlases:
William F. Walker, DSc, ChM, FRCS (Edin. and England), FRS (Edin.).

Single Surgical Procedures 18

A Colour Atlas of

Common Operations on the Foot

Geoffrey Hooper
MMSc, FRCS, FRCSE
*Senior Lecturer in Orthopaedic Surgery,
University of Edinburgh
Honorary Consultant Orthopaedic Surgeon,
Lothian Health Board*

Wolfe Medical Publications Ltd

Dedication

For my father, A. T. Hooper

Copyright © Geoffrey Hooper, 1984
Published by Wolfe Medical Publications Ltd, 1984
Printed by Royal Smeets Offset b.v.,
Weert, Netherlands
ISBN 0 7234 1019 4

ISSN 0264–8695

This book is one of the titles in the series of Wolfe Single Surgical Procedures, a series which will eventually cover some 200 titles.
    If you wish to be kept informed of new additions to the series and receive details of our other titles, please write to Wolfe Medical Publications Ltd, Wolfe House, 3 Conway Street, London W1P 6HE.

All rights reserved. The contents of this book, both photographic and textual, may not be reproduced in any form, by print, photoprint, phototransparency, microfilm, microfiche, or any other means, nor may it be included in any computer retrieval system, without written permission from the publisher.

A few of the other titles in print and in preparation in the Single Surgical Procedures series

Parotidectomy
Traditional Menisectomy
Inguinal Hernias & Hydroceles in Infants and Children
Surgery for Pancreatic & Associated Carcinomata
Subtotal Thyroidectomy
Boari Bladder-Flap Procedure
Treatment of Carpal Tunnel Syndrome
Anterior Resection of Rectum
Seromyotomy for Chronic Duodenal Ulcer
Renal Transplant
Carpal Tunnel Syndrome
Surgery for Undescended Testes
Internal Carotid Artery Surgery
Resection of Aortic Aneurysm
Modified Radical Mastectomy
Discogram Surgery – Lumbar Disc
Total Gastrectomy
Ileo-Rectal Anastomosis
Pre-Prosthetic Oral Surgery
Techniques of Nerve Grafting and Repair
Surgery for Dupuytren's Contracture
Arthrodesis of the Ankle
Surgery for Congenital Dislocation of the Hip
Common Operations on the Foot
Femoral and Tibial Osteotomy
Maxillo-Facial Traumatology
Surgery for Chondromalacia Patellae
Stabilisation for Extensive Spinal Injury
Spondylolisthesis
Laminectomy
Gall Bladder Cholecystectomy
Repair of Prolapsed Rectum
Proctocolectomy
Resection of Oesophagus
Splenectomy
Thyroid Lobectomy
Hirschprung's Disease
Extra-cranial and Intra-cranial Anastomosis
Anterior Nephrectomy
Bladder Augmentation
Caecocystoplasty
Hiatus Hernia
Total Gastrectomy
Billroth 1 Gastrectomy
Billroth 2 Gastrectomy
Abdominal Incisions
Thoracotomy
Chronic Pancreatitis Operation
Surgery for Strictures in Common Bile Duct
Biliary Enteric Anastomosis
Partial Hepatectomy
Splenectomy
Right Hemicolectomy
Appendicectomy
Incisional Hernia
Lung Lobectomy
Lung Removal
Gastric Reconstruction
Surgery for Lymphoedema
Liver Transplant
Pancreas Transplant
Dialysis Techniques
Surgery for Thoracic Outlet
Haemorrhoids
Abdominoperineal Resection of Rectum
Rectosigmoid Resection
Non-resectional Surgery for Multiple Bowel Stenosis
Surgery for Anorectal Incontinence
Craniotomy
Parathyroidectomy
Arterial Injuries
Arterial Bypass Grafts in Leg
Visceral Vascular Occlusion
Varicose Veins Surgery under Local Anaesthesia
Aortofemoral Bypass
Aortoilac Disobliteration
Technique of Small Vessel Repair
Technique of Nerve Grafting and Repair
Microsurgery Techniques
Reimplantation of Ureters

Contents

Acknowledgements	6
Introduction	7
Preparation for operation	9
Arthrodesis of the first metatarsophalangeal joint	13
Arthrodesis of interphalangeal joints	24
Oblique osteotomy of the metatarsal bones	30
Hallux valgus – Keller's arthroplasty	35
Hallux valgus – Mitchell's osteotomy	42
Over-riding fifth toe	51
Plantar interdigital neuroma	56
Ablation of the nail	59
References	62
Index	63

Acknowledgements

I wish to thank Mr Michael Devlin and Mr Graeme Ainslie for their expert photography, Mrs Alison McGowan for typing the manuscript, and the theatre staff of the Princess Margaret Rose Orthopaedic Hospital for their help and patience.

Introduction

The operations that are demonstrated in this book are often performed by surgeons in training. I have deliberately excluded procedures, such as correction of talipes equinovarus or reconstruction of the rheumatoid foot, that should be carried out by more experienced surgeons. I think that it is appropriate in a book of this kind to show only one reliable procedure for each condition, rather than illustrating all the possible procedures and their modifications that have been described. Of course, every surgeon has his own modifications of standard procedures and will pass them on to his trainees, who will in turn devise improvements of their own.

It is fair to say that the results of operations on the foot can be disappointing to both patient and surgeon. There are several reasons for this. It is a mistake to believe that all deformities and painful conditions of the foot require surgical treatment. An operation should be recommended only when there is a reasonable expectation, based on the surgeon's experience, that it will be of benefit to the patient; there is no place for the 'try it and see' approach. Many patients have unrealistic expectations of surgical treatment. They may not know that it can take several weeks for the foot to settle down after operation and that they will not feel the benefit of the operation for some time. The time spent discussing the aims of the operation and postoperative management is never wasted.

General conditions such as diabetes or peripheral vascular disease may preclude operation; therefore a careful general assessment of the patient before operation is most important.

Successful results depend on:
(a) Careful selection of patients;
(b) Performing the appropriate operation for the individual patient's problem;
(c) Careful surgical technique and postoperative management.

Note
Because the diameters of malleable surgical wire and stiff Kirschner wires are expressed by their manufacturers in Standard Wire Gauge and inches respectively, I have kept to these units in this book. Other measurements are given in metric units. I apologise for this inconsistency.

Preparation for operation

It is of utmost importance that the patient's identity and the side of operation is checked with the patient before induction of anaesthesia. The foot or digit involved should have been marked with ink in the ward, but should always be confirmed with the patient and checked against the notes.

General anaesthesia is recommended for the procedures described in this book. After induction a pneumatic tourniquet is applied above the knee and inflated after the limb has been exsanguinated with an Esmarch bandage. The time of application is noted. If identical procedures are to be carried out on both feet, tourniquets are placed on both legs before draping. None of the operations described takes more than a few minutes to perform, so there should be no risk of leaving the tourniquet on for longer than is safe. However, to shorten tourniquet time two teams can work simultaneously. Alternatively, one tourniquet is inflated and released after the first operation has been completed; the tourniquet on the other leg is then inflated after exsanguinating the leg with a sterile Esmarch bandage.

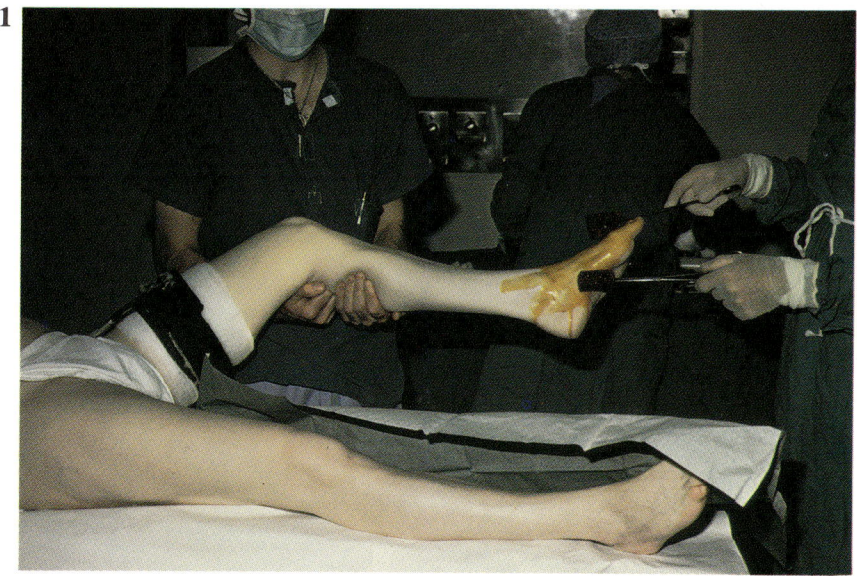

1 Skin preparation. An assistant supports the leg and the skin is prepared using two sponges in holders. One is used to paint the foot and the other to stabilise it.

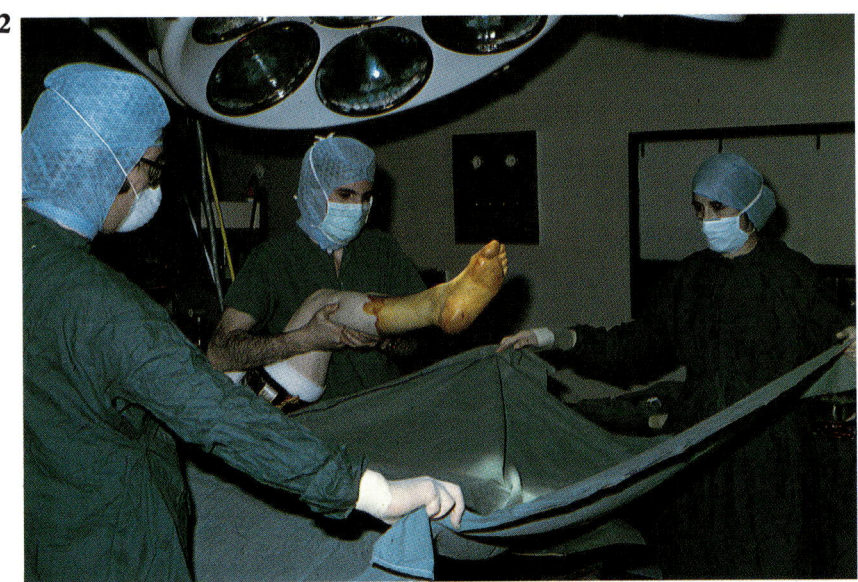

2 A large drape is placed beneath the leg on which the procedure is to be carried out.

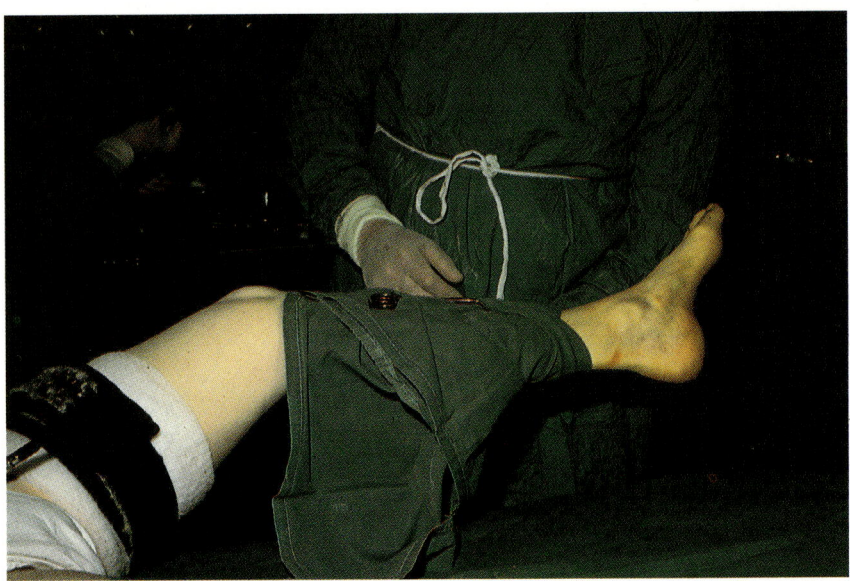

3 A small drape, folded to a triangle, is clipped around the ankle and the leg is lowered to rest on the table.

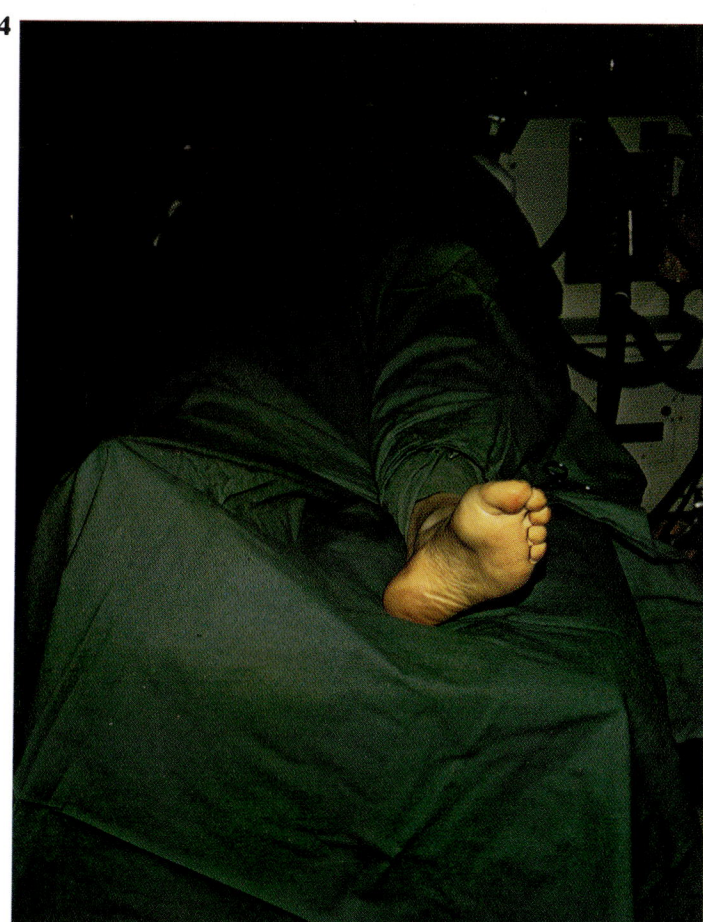

4 A further large drape is used to cover the patient and is clipped around the ankle.

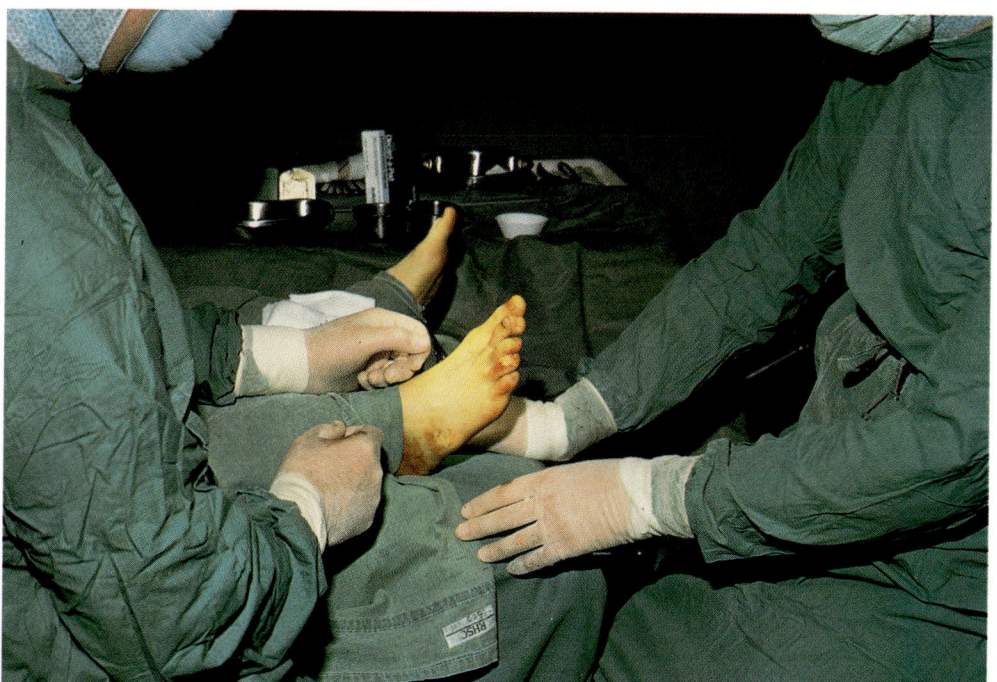

5 Ready to start. The surgeon and his assistant are sitting, the surgeon facing the field of the operation.

6 · On completion of the operation 3 to 5 ml of plain 0.5 per cent bupivacaine hydrochloride is infiltrated into the wound or instilled into it before closure. This provides excellent postoperative analgesia for several hours.

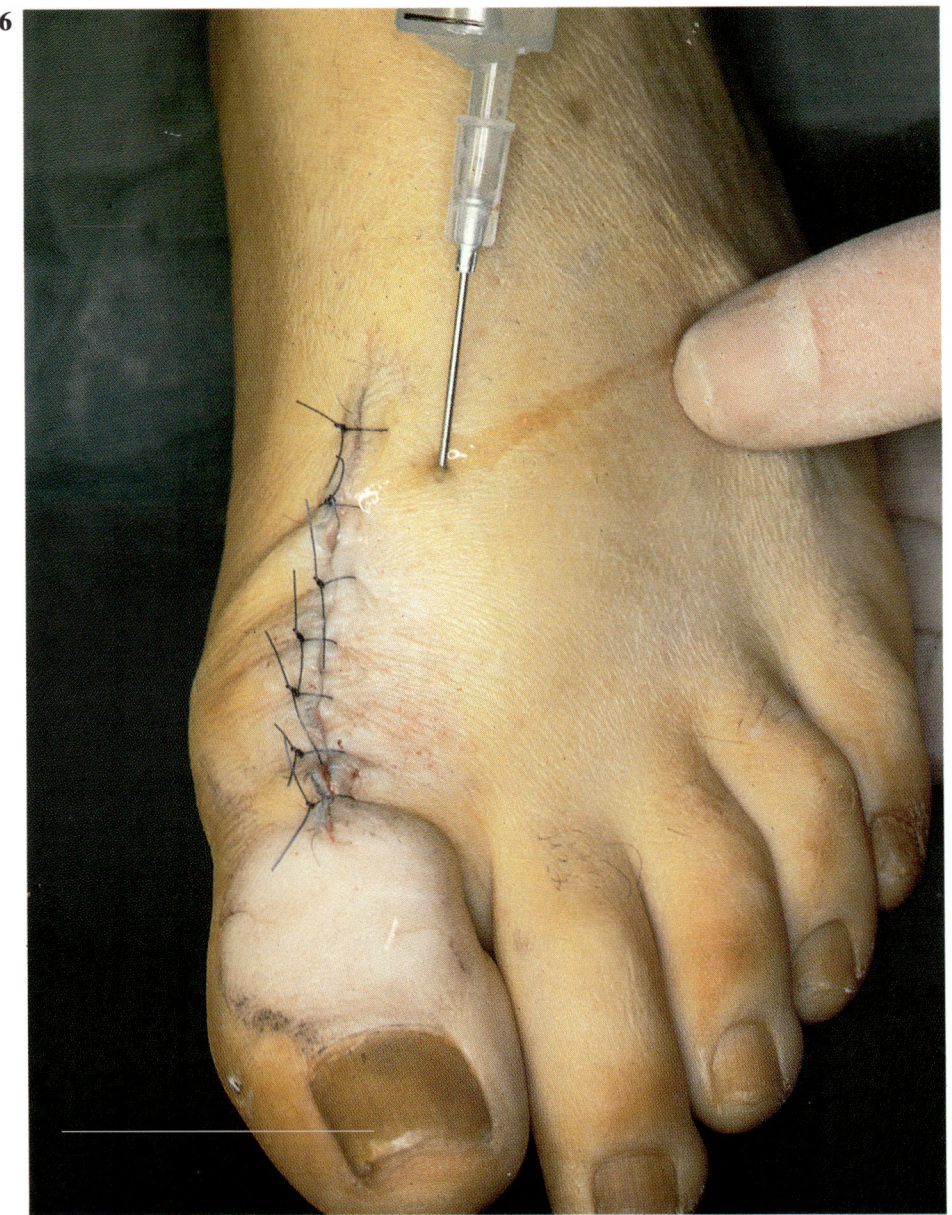

Arthrodesis of the first metatarsophalangeal joint

The most common indication for this procedure is in the treatment of hallux rigidus (osteoarthrosis of the first metatarsophalangeal joint). In established hallux rigidus the toe is flexed at the metatarsophalangeal joint and a dorsal osteophyte is visible and palpable (see **7**). Because dorsiflexion is limited or absent (see **9**) pain is experienced in the 'toe-off' position of the gait cycle.

The aim of the operation is to fuse the joint in about 10 to 15 degrees of dorsiflexion, or slightly more if the patient prefers a raised heel on the shoe. The operation is contraindicated if there are degenerative changes in the interphalangeal joint of the big toe.

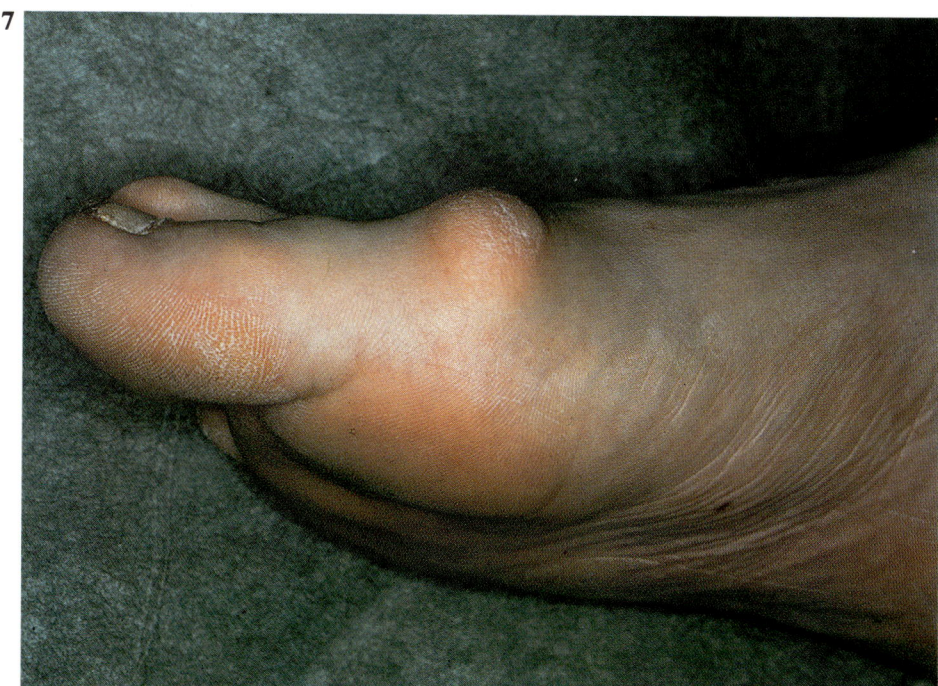

7 Hallux rigidus. There is often a dorsal osteophyte and a flexion deformity at the metatarsophalangeal joint.

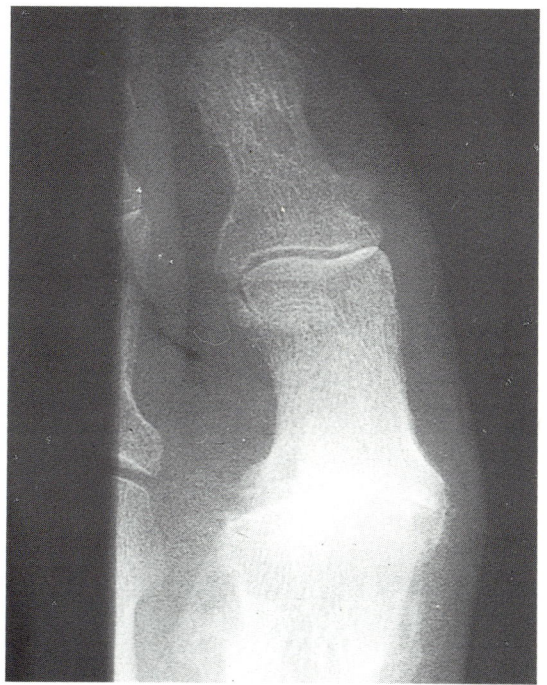

8 Radiographic appearance, showing marked degenerative changes in a case of hallux rigidus.

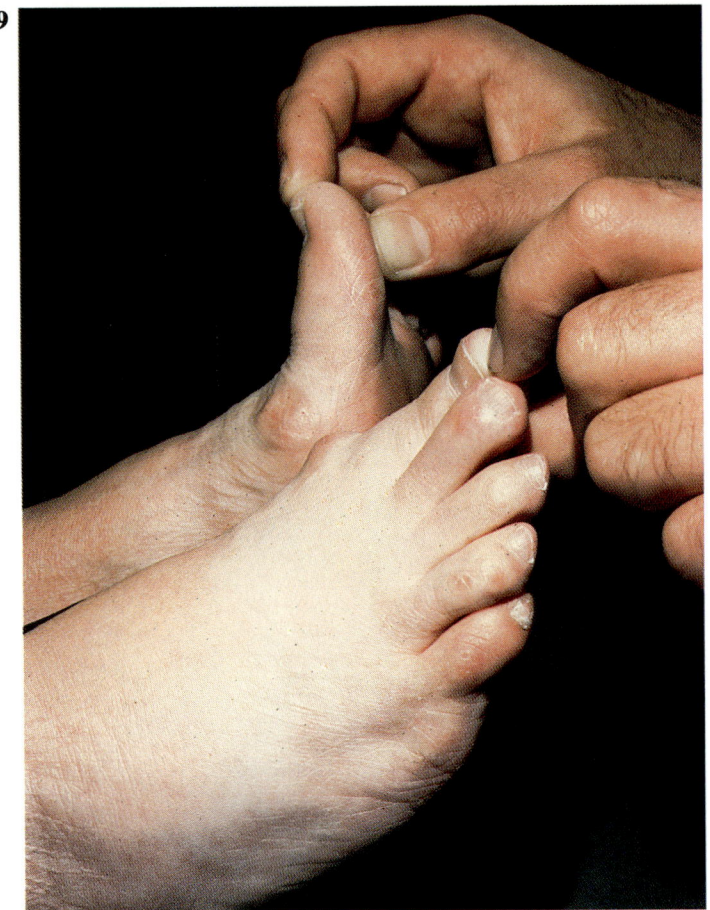 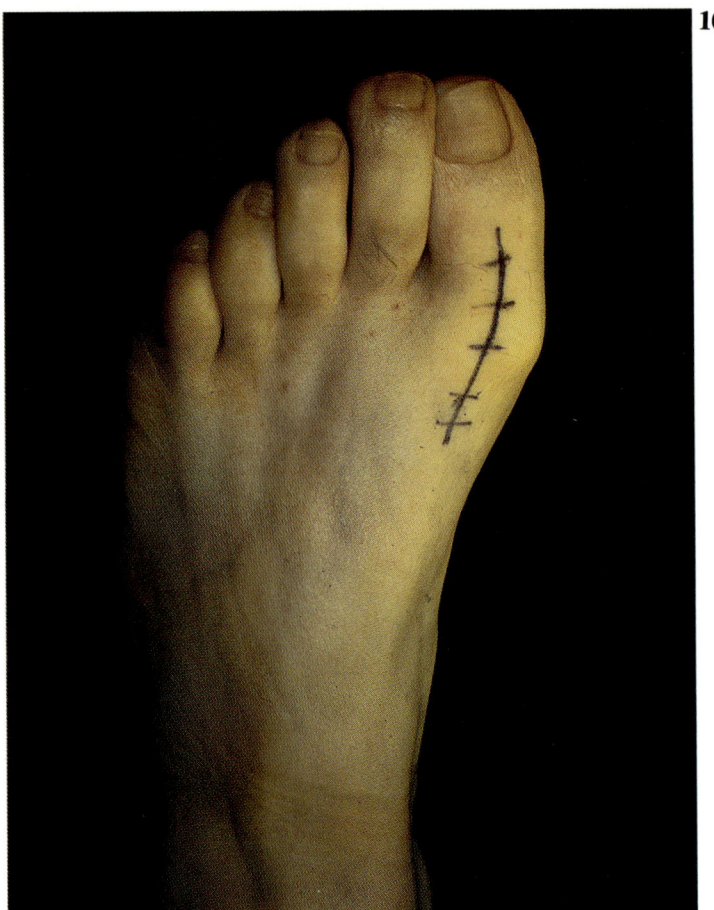

9 Dorsiflexion is limited or absent. In this patient the right great toe is affected.

10 A slightly curved dorsal incision is centred over the joint, to the medial side of the tendon of extensor hallucis longus. The incision should not lie over the tendon, or else uncomfortable adhesions may develop.

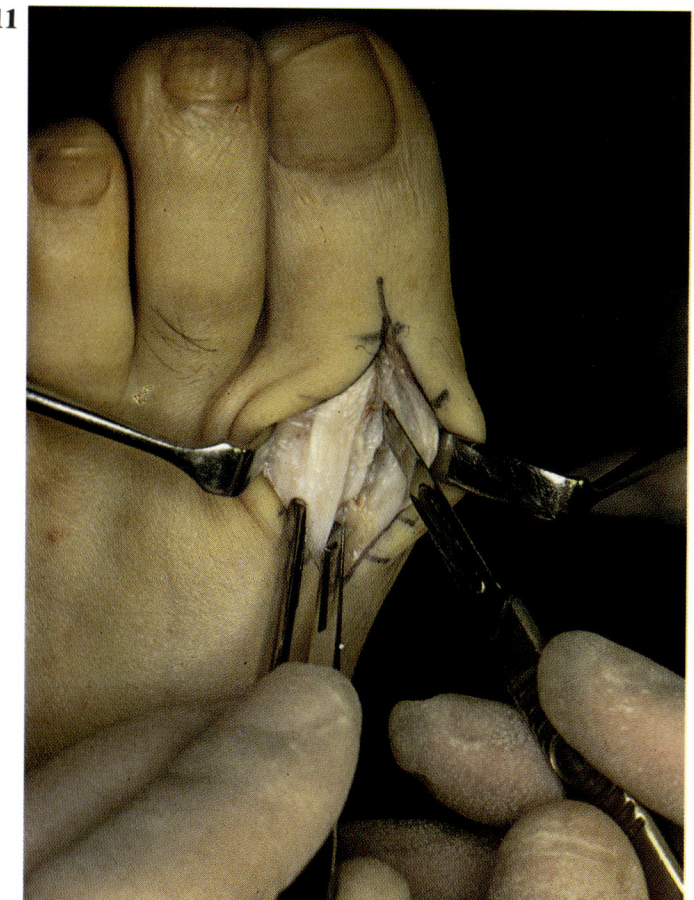
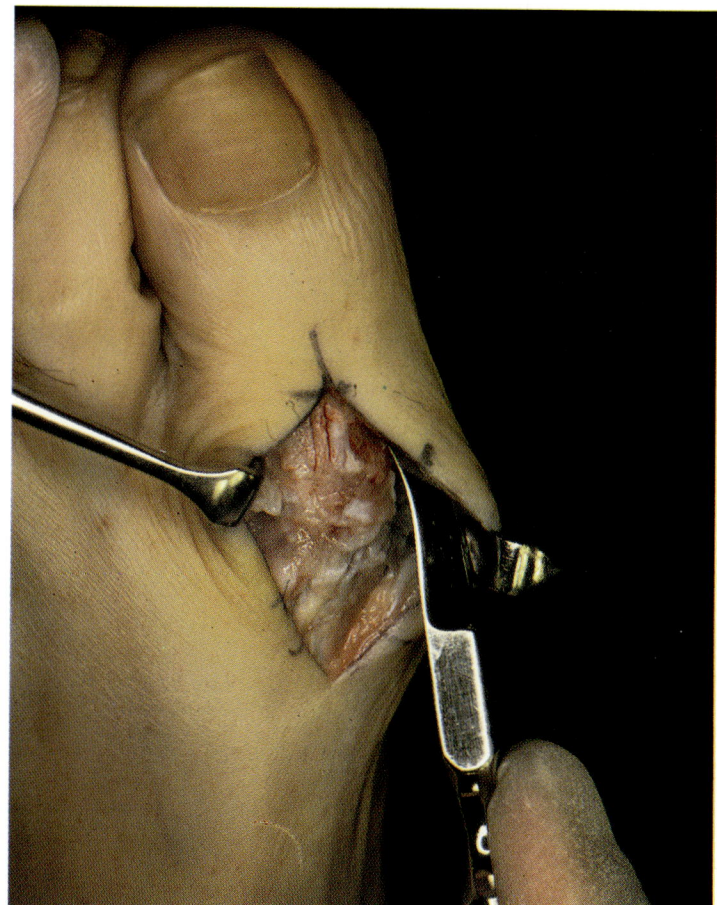

11 After coagulating small veins the incision is deepened to bone, protecting the tendon of extensor hallucis longus.

12 A periosteal elevator is used to raise the soft tissues from the head and neck of the metatarsal bone and the proximal half of the proximal phalanx.

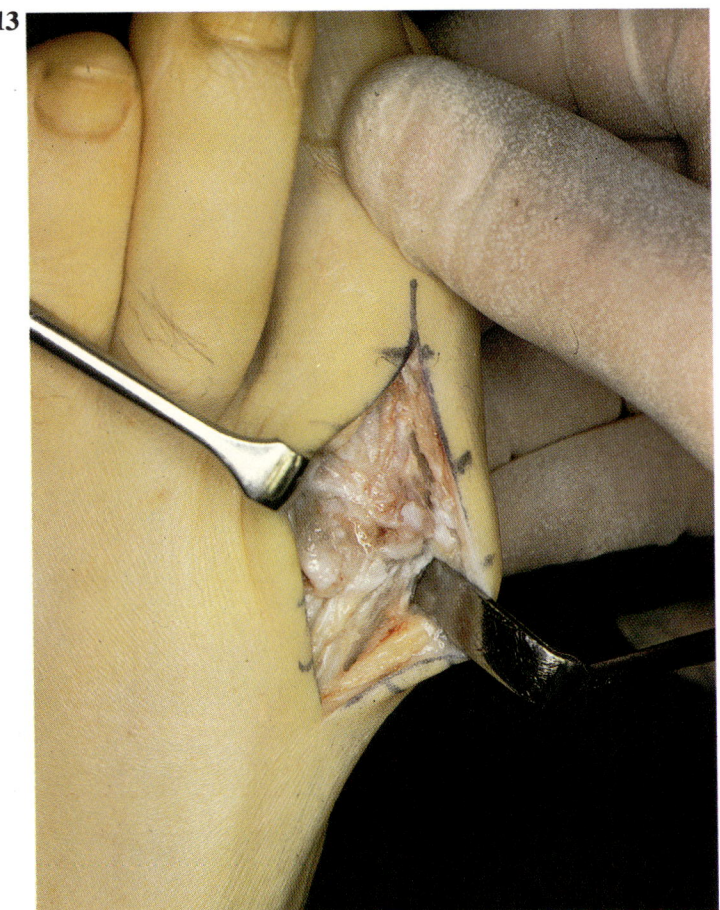
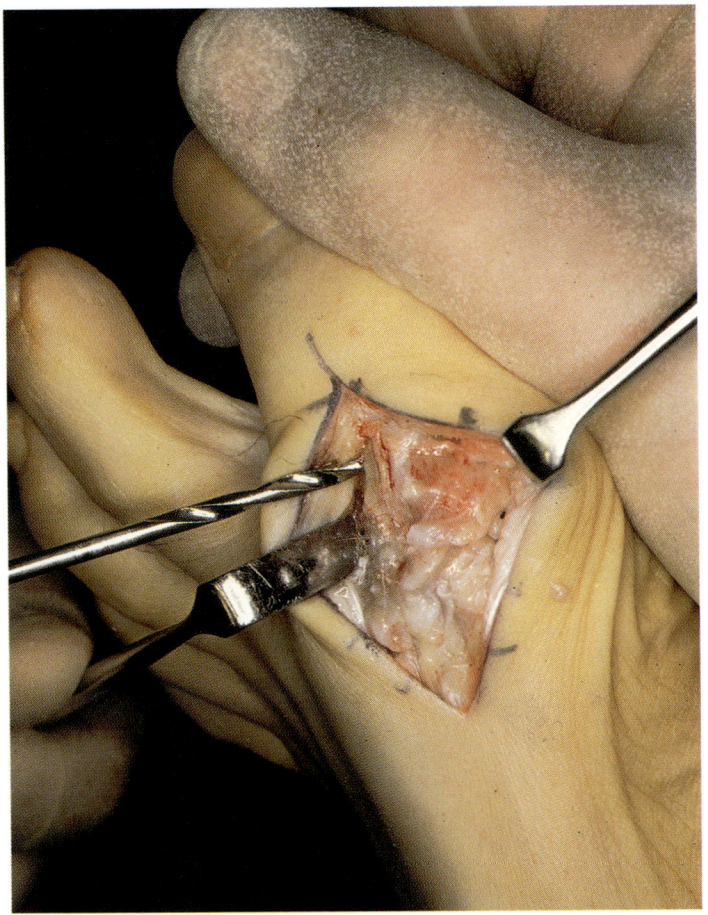

13 When the remains of the joint capsule have been removed the joint can be opened widely to expose the remains of the articular surfaces.

14 Using a 2 mm drill two parallel holes are drilled in the metatarsal neck and the proximal phalanx, each being about 1.5 cm from the joint. The holes should lie in the transverse plane to make later retrieval of the ends of the wire easier (see **15**), but the exact plane is not important, so long as they are parallel.

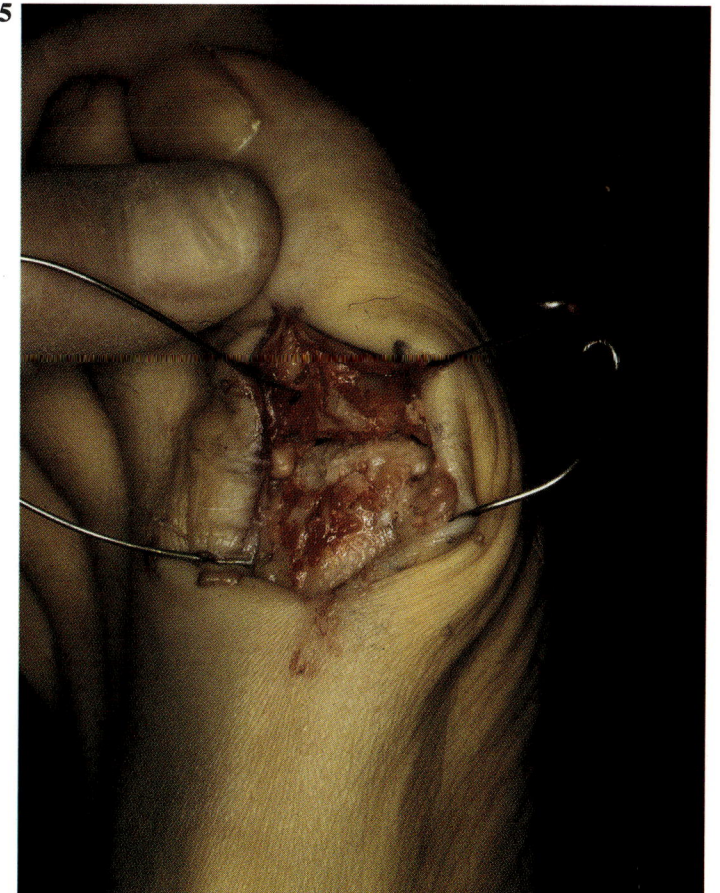
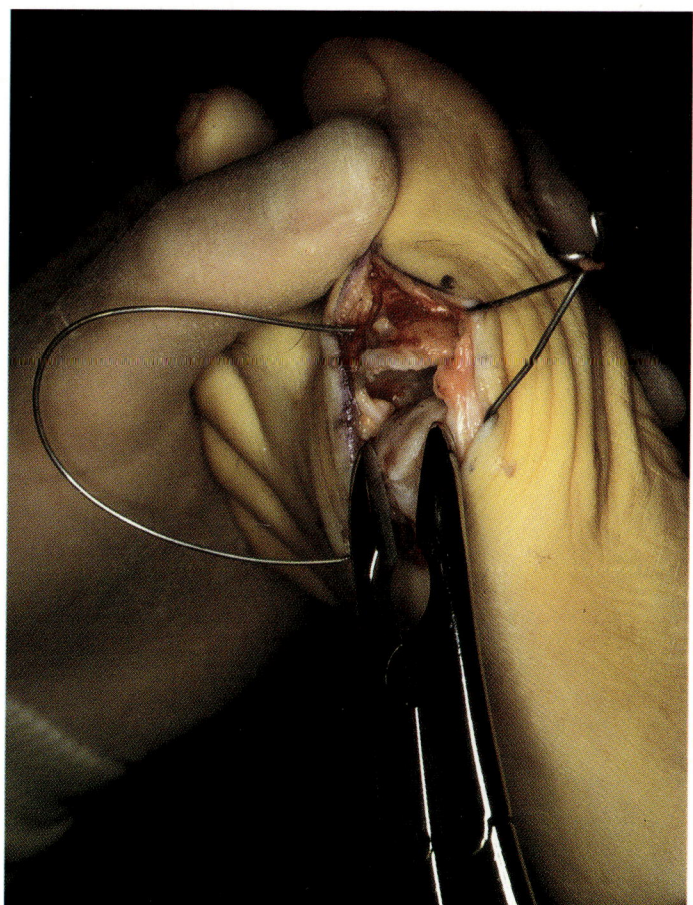

15 A loop of 20 swg wire is passed through the holes. It is not important if the ends lie medially (as shown) or laterally, provided they are buried carefully at the end of the procedure.

16 Using bone nibbling forceps dorsal osteophytes are removed and the residual articular cartilage and subchondral bone is removed from the metatarsal head.

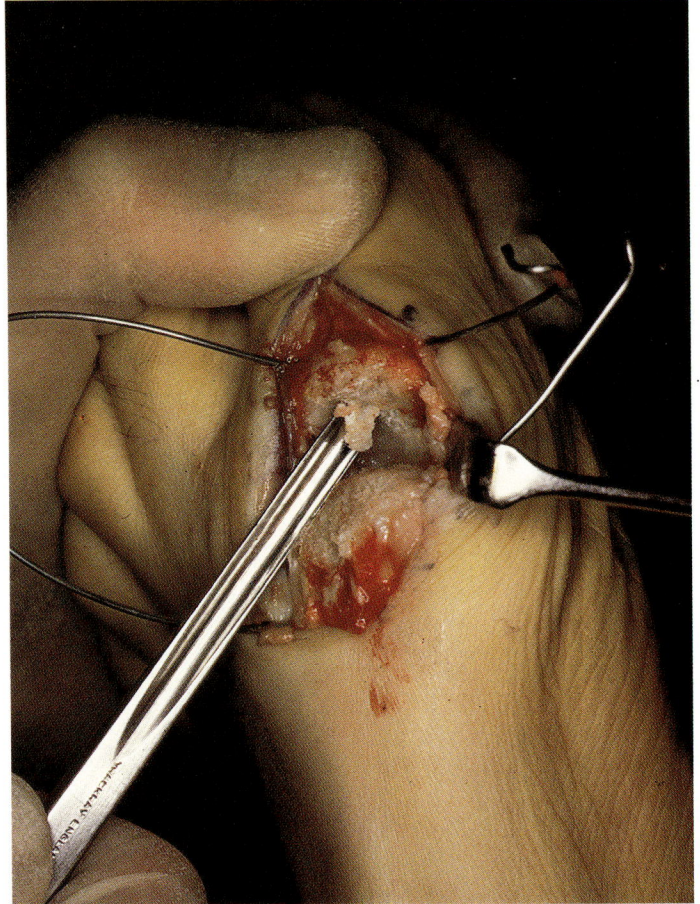

17 Gouges and nibbling forceps are used to remove articular cartilage and subchondral bone from the base of the proximal phalanx. This bone can be very hard and patience is absolutely necessary. A successful arthrodesis is dependent upon exposing cancellous bone on the surfaces to be placed in apposition.

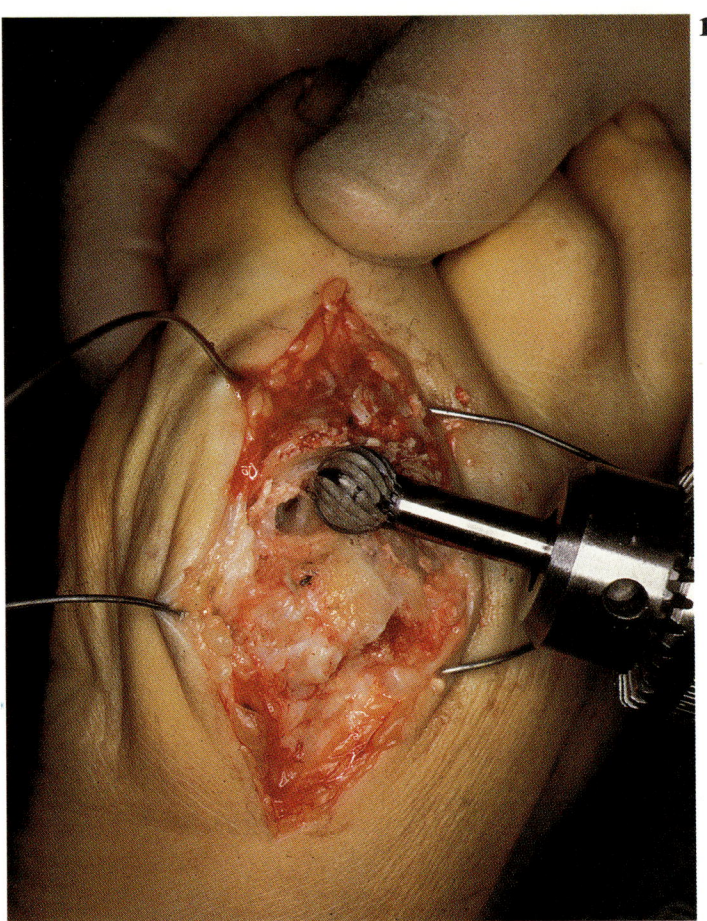

18 A power-driven burr will save time and effort at this stage of the operation.

19 The convexity of the metatarsal head should make good contact with the base of the proximal phalanx. If the surfaces do not fit, more bone is removed as appropriate. A few drill holes are made in the opposing surfaces to help break up the hard subchondral bone and facilitate removal of bone with nibbling forceps.

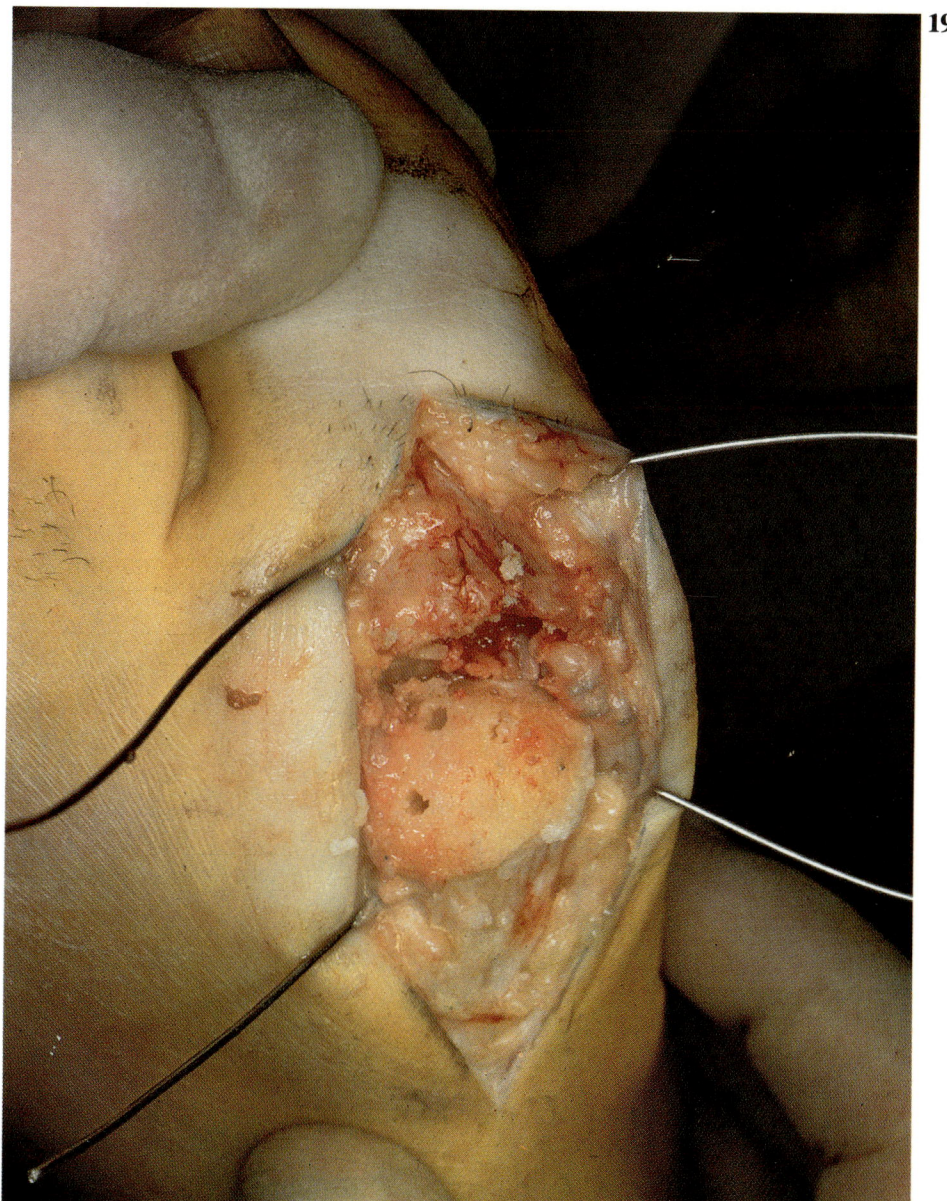

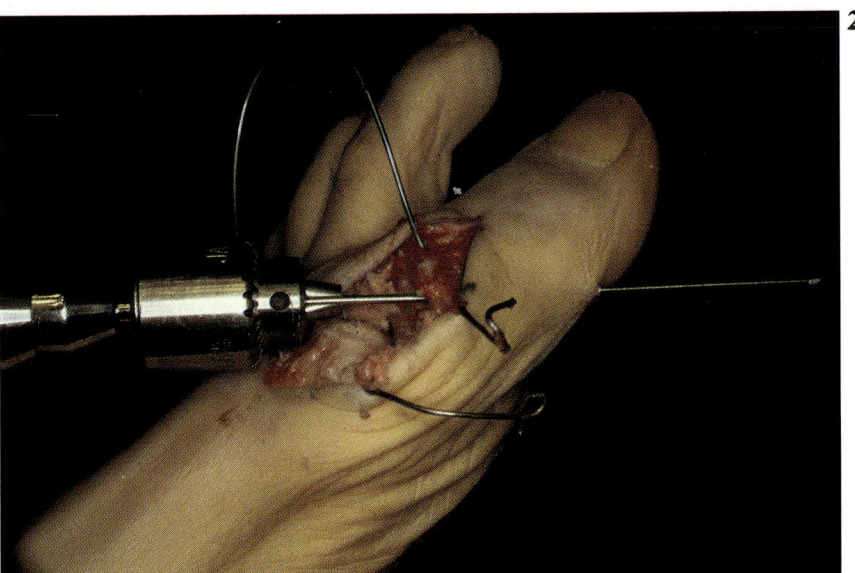

20 and 21 A 0.062″ double-ended Kirschner wire about 15 cm long is driven obliquely from the joint into the proximal phalanx, using a power drill. It should leave the bone just proximal to the interphalangeal joint (see **25**) and be inserted at such an angle that it can be driven back in the metatarsal bone for a reasonable depth. The desired direction is first estimated by laying a wire on the skin.

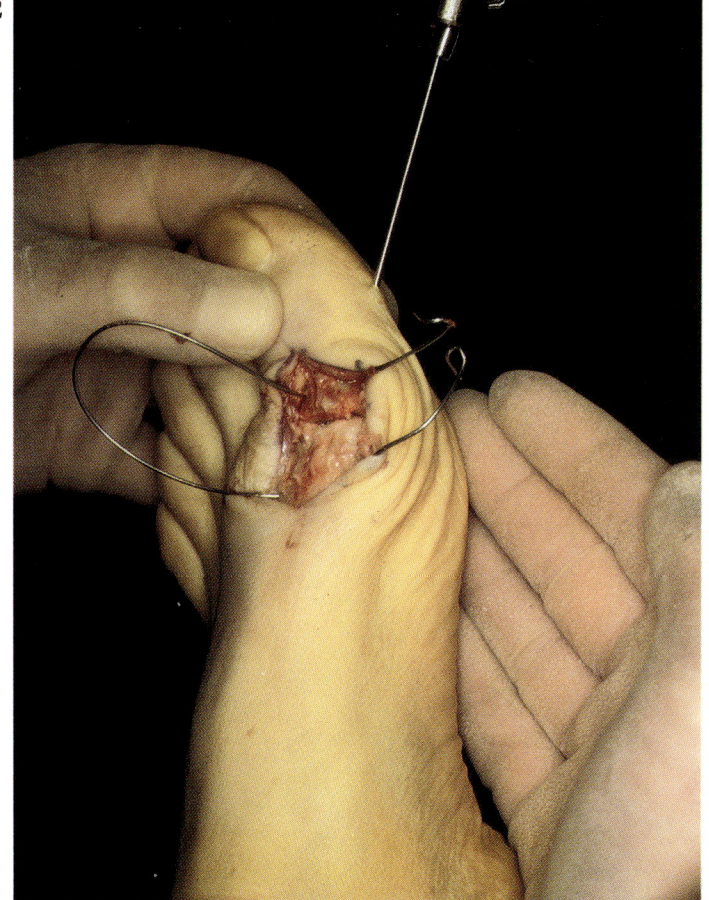

22 The wire is driven retrograde into the metatarsal bone after it has been withdrawn into the proximal phalanx sufficiently to allow the bone surfaces to be opposed. The desired position of the great toe (10 to 15 degrees of dorsiflexion, 15 to 20 degrees of valgus and no rotation) should be obtained before the wire is driven retrograde. After inserting the wire the position is checked again and if it is unsatisfactory the wire is withdrawn and reinserted.

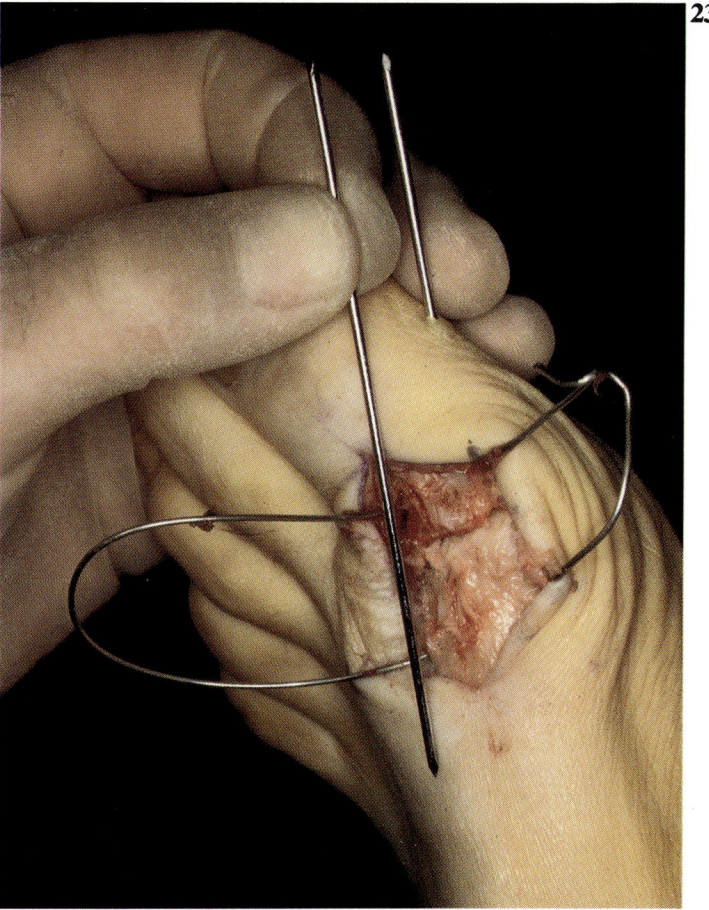

23 Another K-wire of the same length is used to check the angle and depth of penetration into the metatarsal bone.

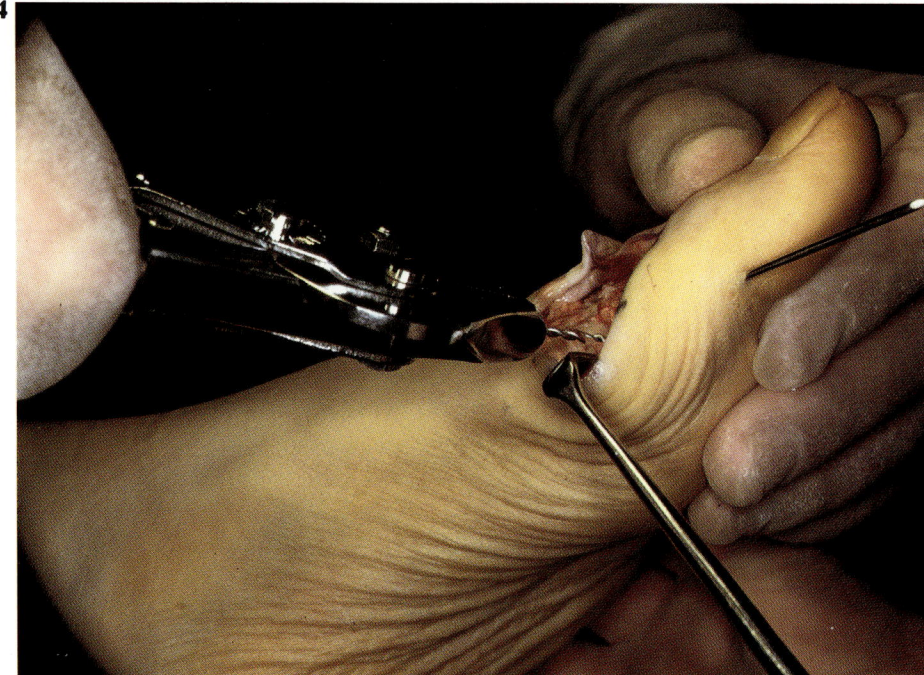

24 The wire loop is tightened with pliers. The ends of the wire loop are cut off leaving a 1 cm length of twisted wire which is turned to lie flat on the bone and buried beneath soft tissue away from the suture line. The K-wire is cut leaving about 2 mm protruding from the skin. Skin is closed with 3–0 interrupted nylon sutures and bupivacaine is infiltrated into the wound.

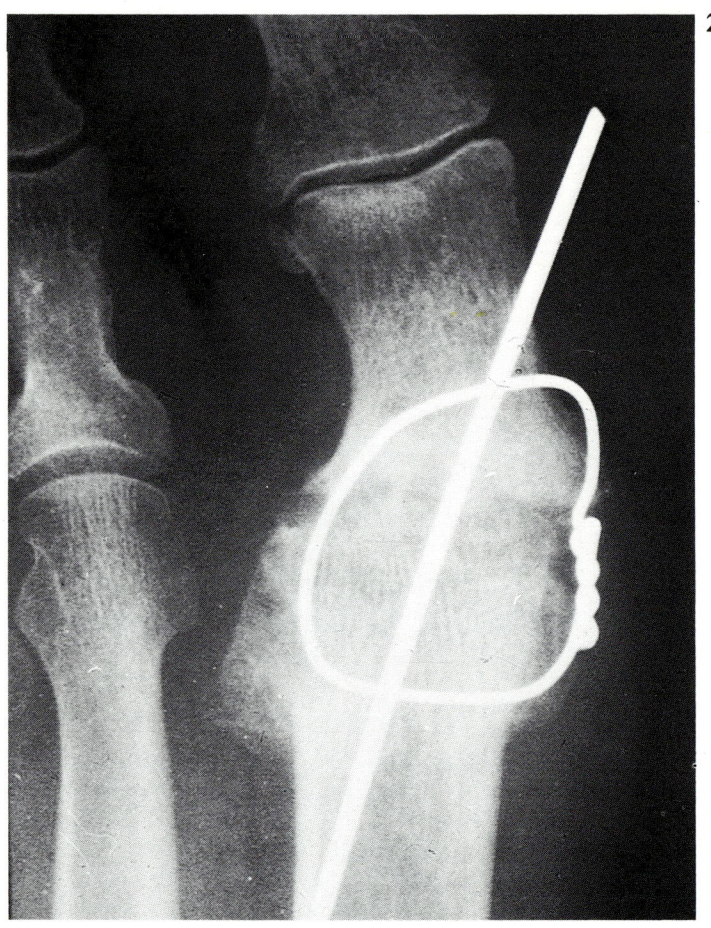

25 The postoperative radiographic appearance.

Postoperative management

A light wool and crepe bandage is applied in the operating theatre. The patient keeps the foot elevated for 2 or 3 days; after this period a below-knee plaster with walking rocker and protective toe extension is applied. Although limited walking is allowed, the patient should keep the foot elevated as much as possible for the first week or two to prevent swelling. Stitches are removed 14 days after operation. The plaster is retained for six weeks. On removal of the plaster the K-wire can be removed if the radiographic appearance of the arthrodesis is satisfactory. The K-wire can be withdrawn with pliers without difficulty or discomfort; it is not necessary to remove the wire loop. If the arthrodesis feels solid, the patient may return to wearing a normal shoe.

Complications

Postoperative swelling is kept to a minimum by elevation of the foot.

Haematoma formation is uncommon if skin vessels have been coagulated.

Infection should also be uncommon, but if it occurs it is treated by elevation of the foot and the use of antibiotics.

Non-union. This has not been a problem with the technique described but if it occurred the operation could be repeated, taking care to remove the bone surfaces down to cancellous bone and possibly adding a cancellous bone graft.

Malposition of the big toe will cause painful pressure on the toe from the shoe. It should not occur with the technique described because it is simple to carry out minor adjustments of the position of the great toe before completing the operation.

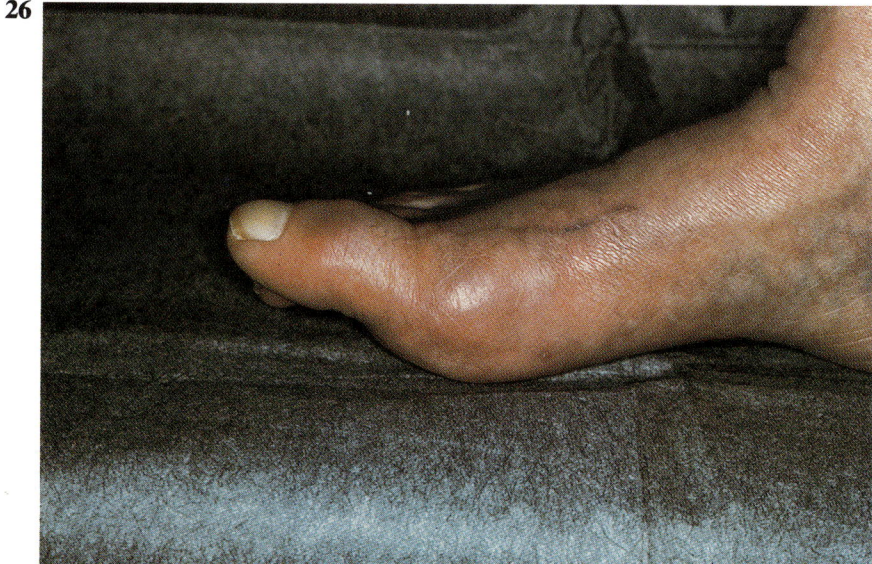

26 Malposition of the toe in dorsiflexion after arthrodesis.

Arthrodesis of interphalangeal joints

Arthrodesis of one or other of the interphalangeal joints is indicated when a mallet or hammer toe deformity causes the formation of painful callosities. Arthrodesis of a distal interphalangeal joint will be illustrated.

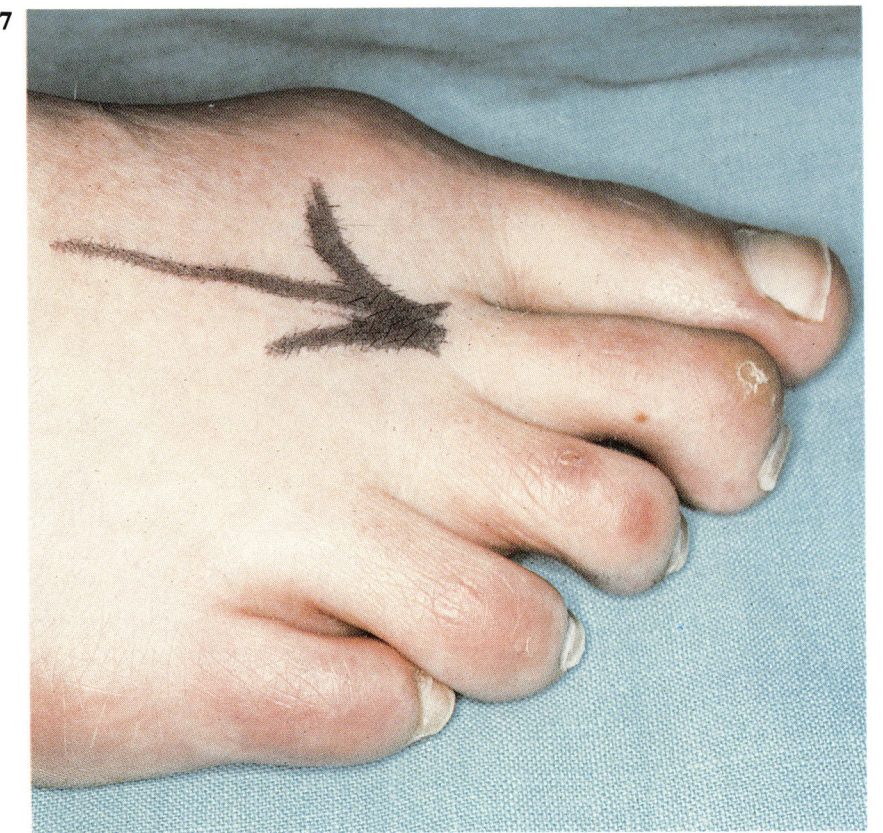

27 Mallet toe. There is a flexion deformity of the distal interphalangeal (DIP) joint. A callosity forms on the pulp of the toe and the nail may be deformed. There is often a callosity over the DIP joint.

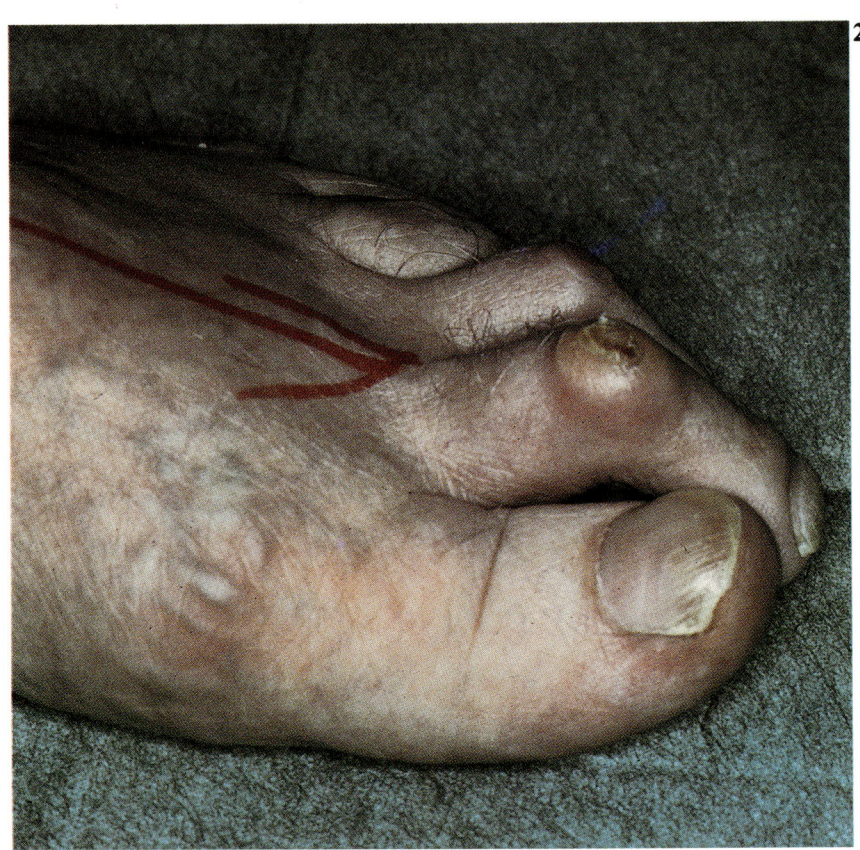

28 Hammer toe. There is a flexion deformity of the proximal interphalangeal (PIP) joint and a hyperextension deformity of the distal joint. There is a dorsal callosity over the PIP joint.

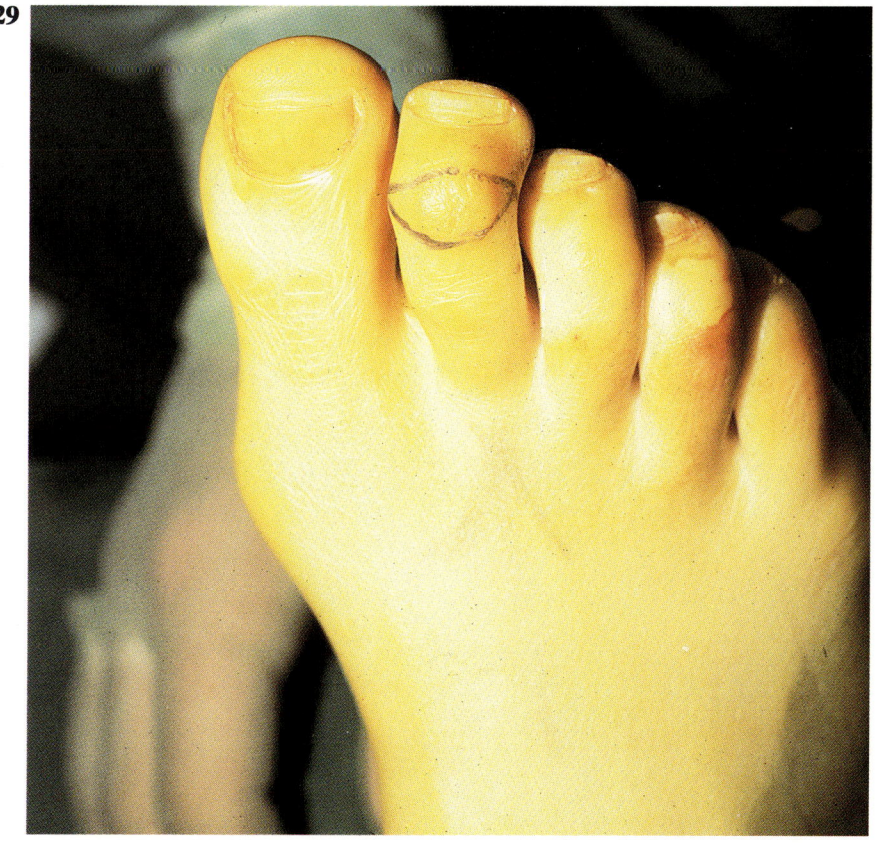

29 An elliptical incision around the callosity is marked out over the DIP joint.

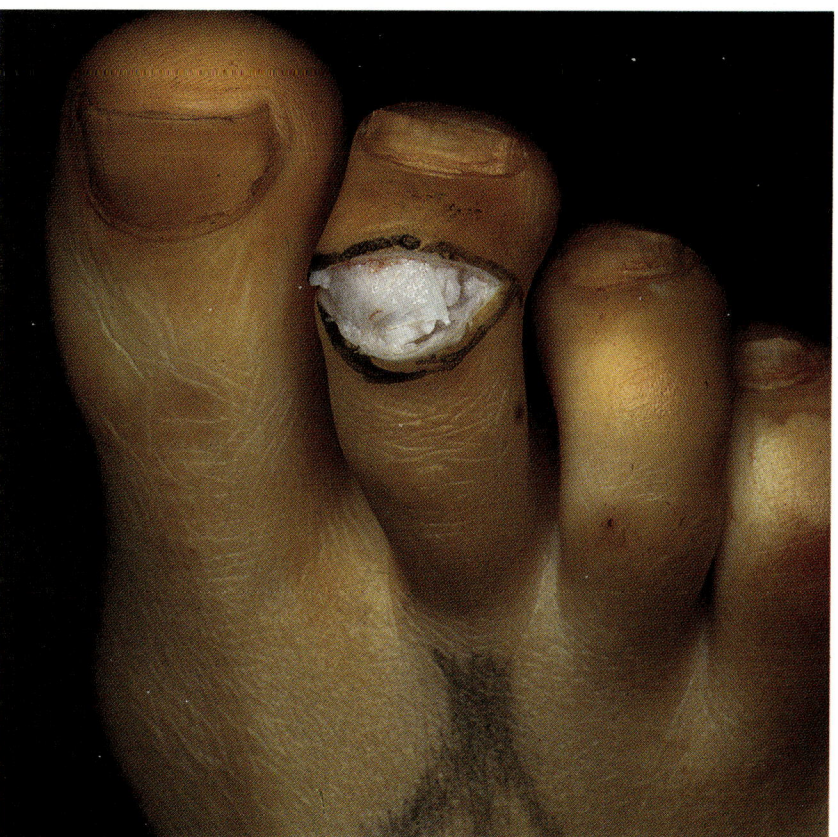

30 The ellipse of skin is removed to expose the extensor tendon.

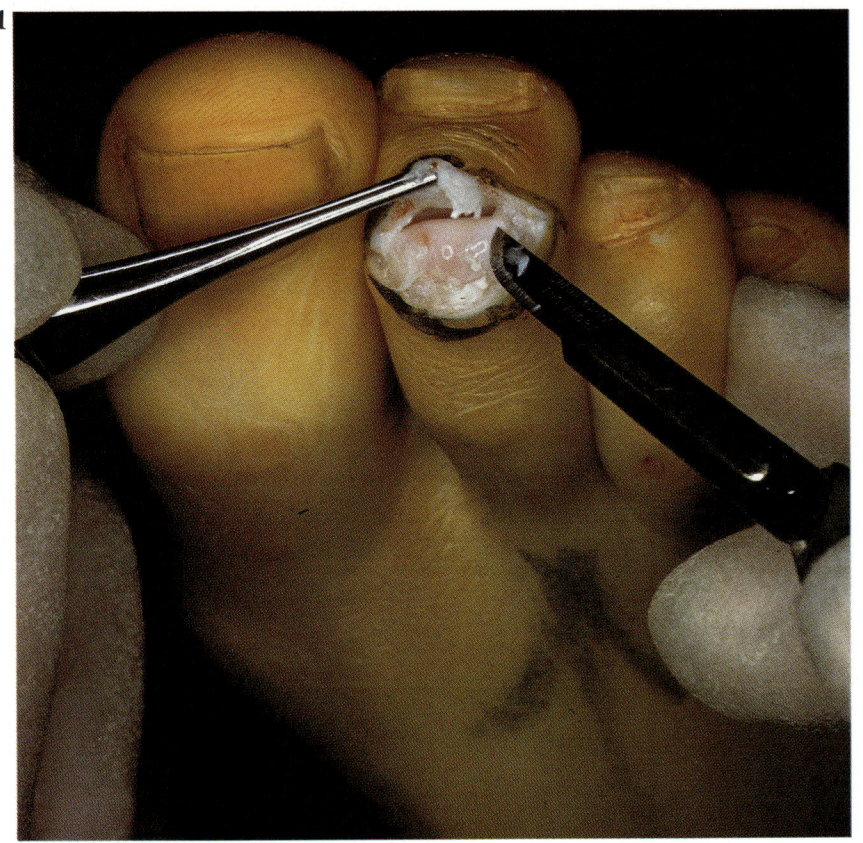

31 The joint is opened using a knife to excise the extensor tendon and dorsal capsule. The collateral ligaments are divided to allow the joint to be opened widely, but the plantar aspect of the joint is not disturbed.

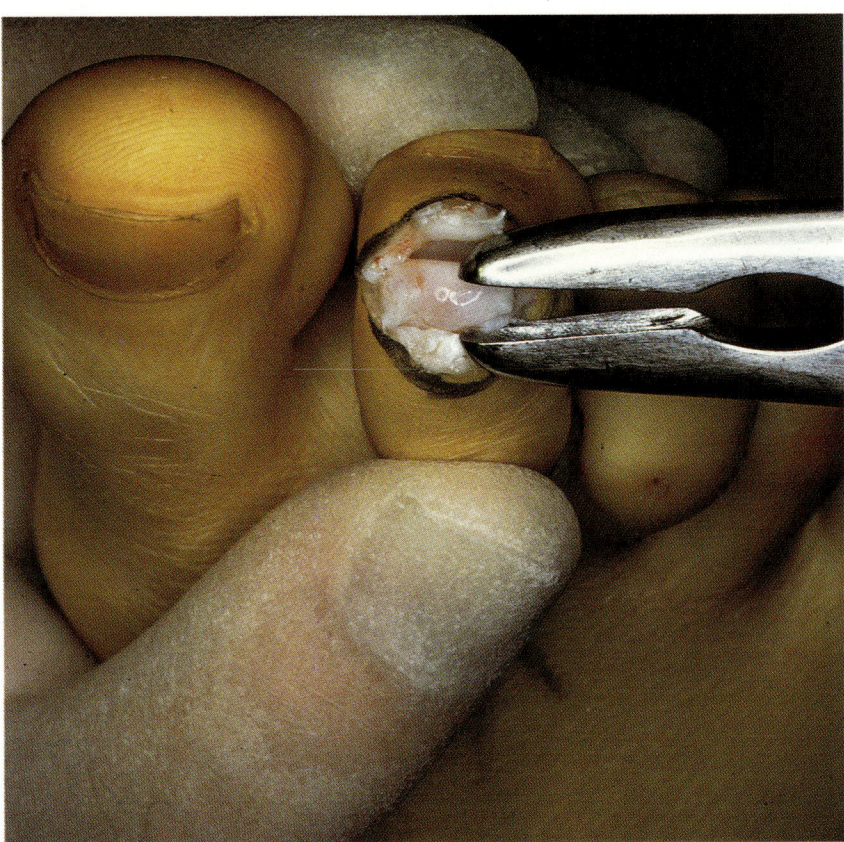

32 Small bone-nibbling forceps are used to remove the articular surfaces down to cancellous bone.

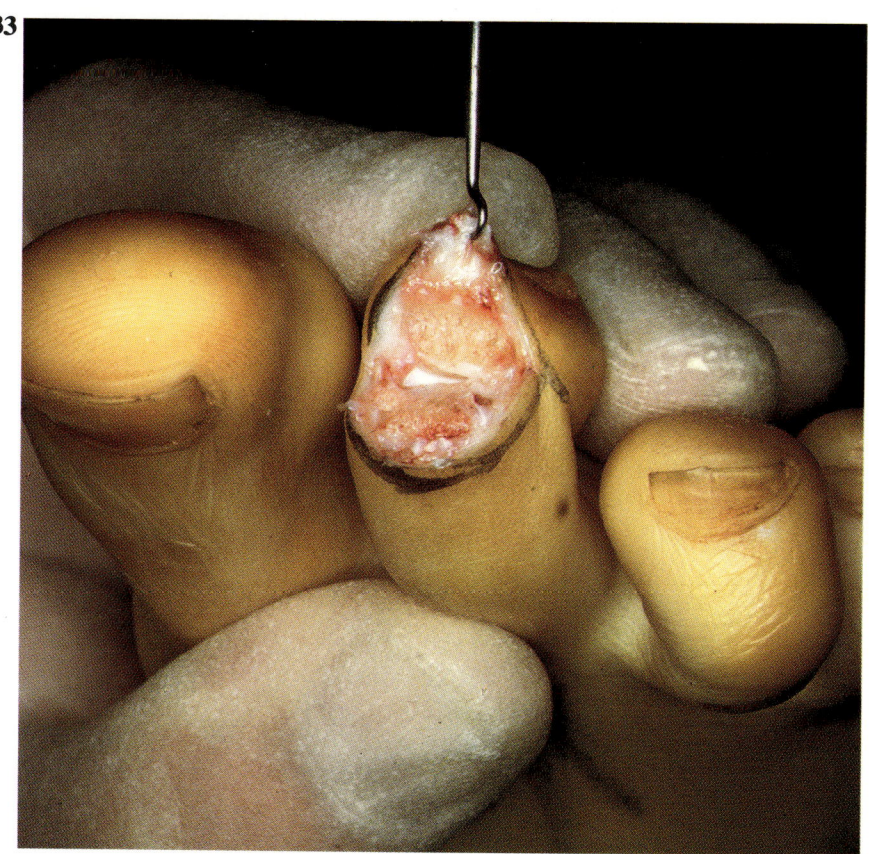

33 The contours of the articular surfaces are retained, allowing the convexity of the head of the intermediate phalanx to fit snugly into the concavity at the base of the terminal phalanx.

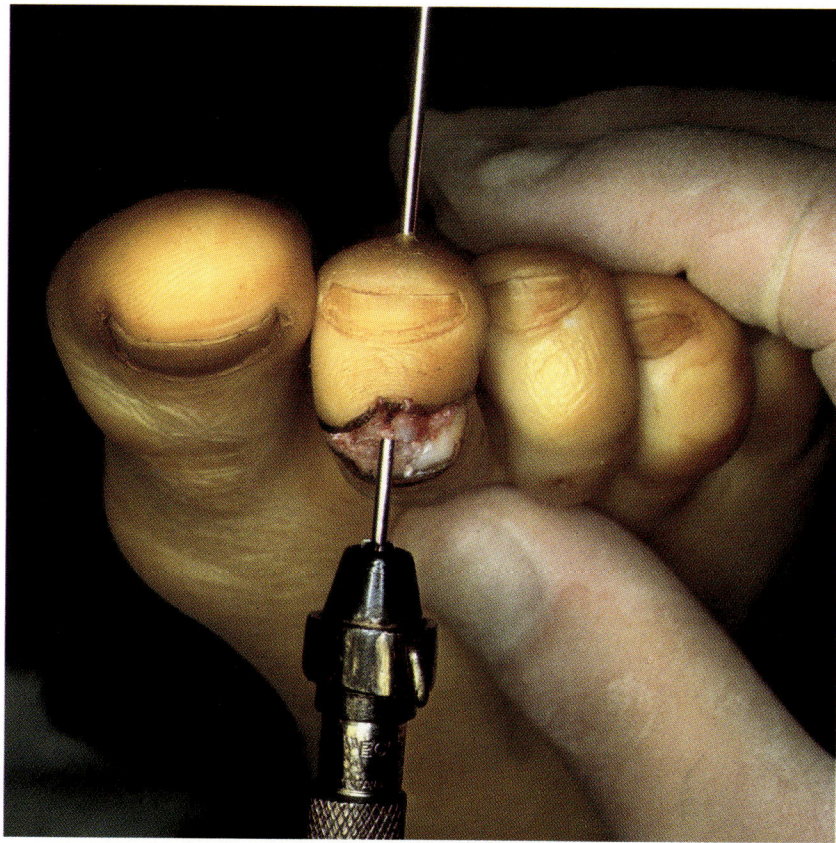

34 A 0.045" diameter double-ended Kirschner wire is driven from the joint out of the end of the toe using a hand or power drill.

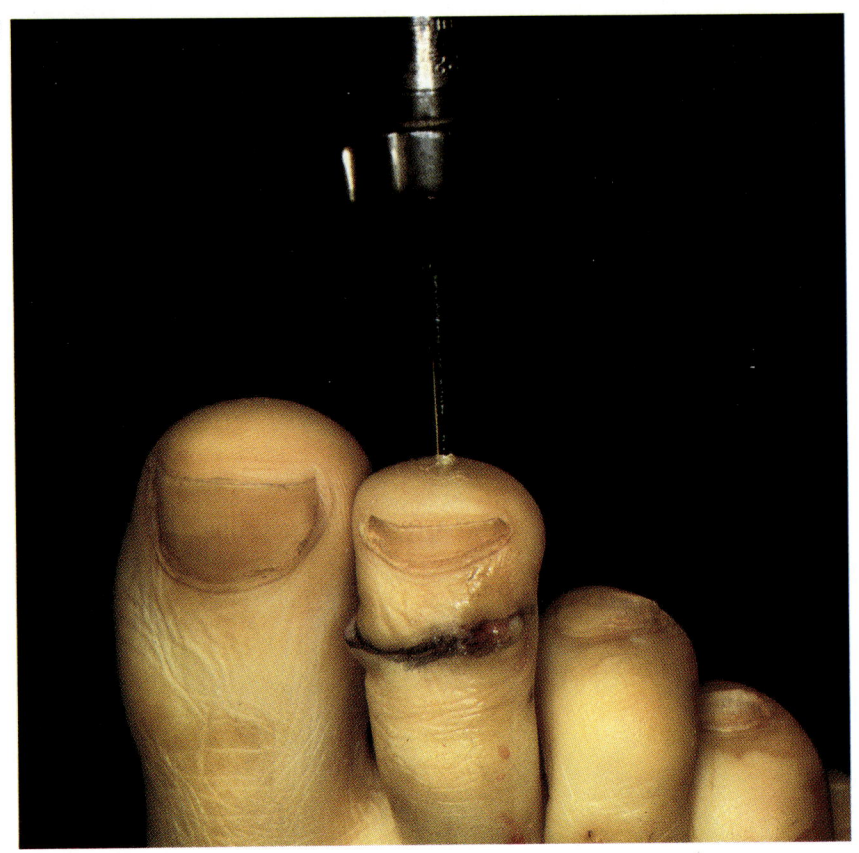

35 **The joint is then stabilised by driving the wire back along the toe,** after checking that the bone ends fit snugly.

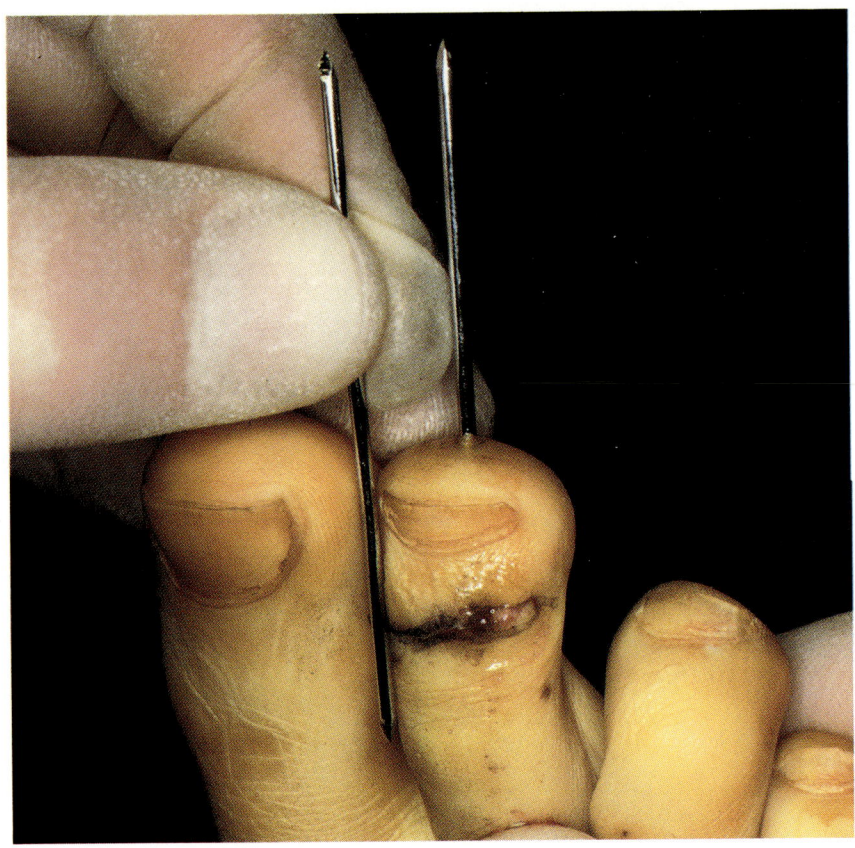

36 **The position of the K-wire is checked using an identical wire.** It should be driven about 2 cm into the toe past the joint. It does not matter if it crosses the PIP joint.

37 The K-wire is cut short. The end can be bent over, as shown here, or protected with the soft plastic seal from the plunger of a disposable syringe. It should not be cut flush with the skin or it may be difficult to remove. The extensor tendon and the skin are closed with a couple of absorbable (Dexon or Vicryl) sutures that pick up both layers. Bupivacaine is infiltrated around the base of the toe.

Postoperative management

A light gauze dressing is placed around the toe. Circulation in the toe is checked carefully after removal of the tourniquet. Often the dressing will harden with dried blood and this makes a satisfactory 'plaster', but a more aesthetic arrangement is to apply a collodion soaked dressing when any swelling of the toes has gone down. Walking should be restricted for a week or two and the patient told to keep the foot elevated. The dressing and K-wire are removed six weeks after operation. The arthrodesis is usually solid but if not the fibrous union is usually very stable and pain free.

Complications

The circulation in the toe can be compromised by damage to the digital arteries if the plantar part of the capsule is cut, or by compression resulting from tight dressings. These complications can be readily avoided by careful dissection, avoiding the application of tight bandages and regularly checking the circulation after operation. All dressings should be removed if the circulation is suspect.

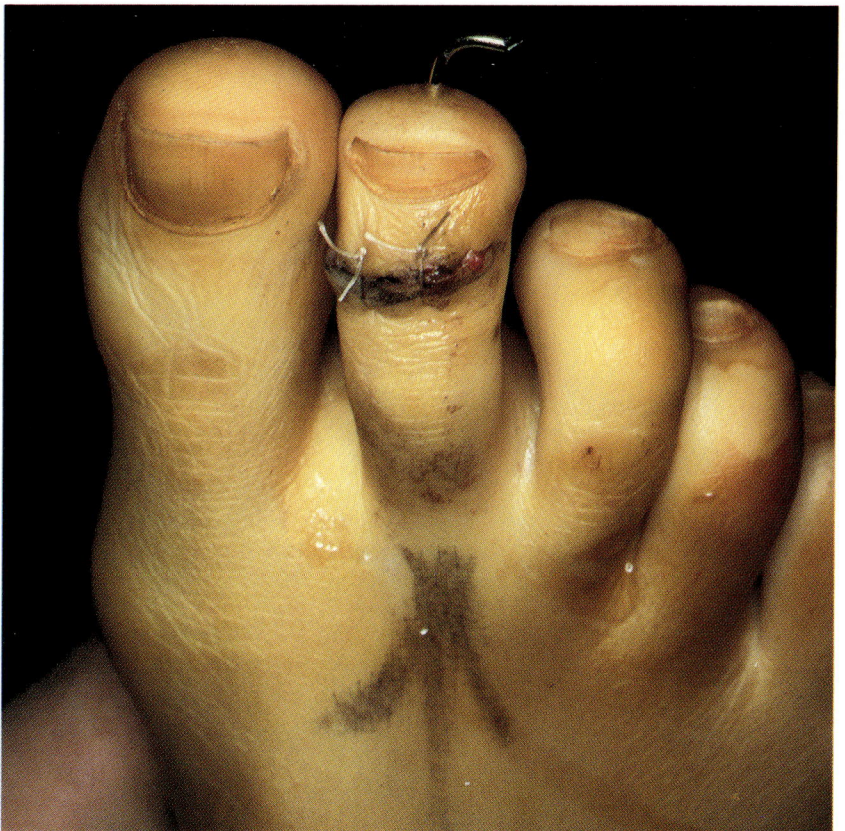

Oblique osteotomy of the metatarsal bones — Helal's operation

Metatarsalgia may be caused by prominence of one or more metatarsal heads in the sole of the foot. It is a common clinical condition in middle-age, associated with spreading out of the anterior part of the foot and stiffness in the tarsometatarsal joints. A tender callosity forms under the involved metatarsal head.

38 A callosity in the sole beneath the second metatarsal head. There is also a severe hallux valgus deformity which will also be corrected (see **45 to 58**). Metatarsalgia and hallux valgus are frequently associated; it is important to realise that the complaint of metatarsalgia will not be helped by surgical treatment of the hallux valgus.

The aim of metatarsal osteotomy is to realign the head of the appropriate metatarsal bone (usually the second) and thus relieve pressure on the callosity when walking. It can be combined with other operations on the foot, for example, correction of a hallux valgus deformity.

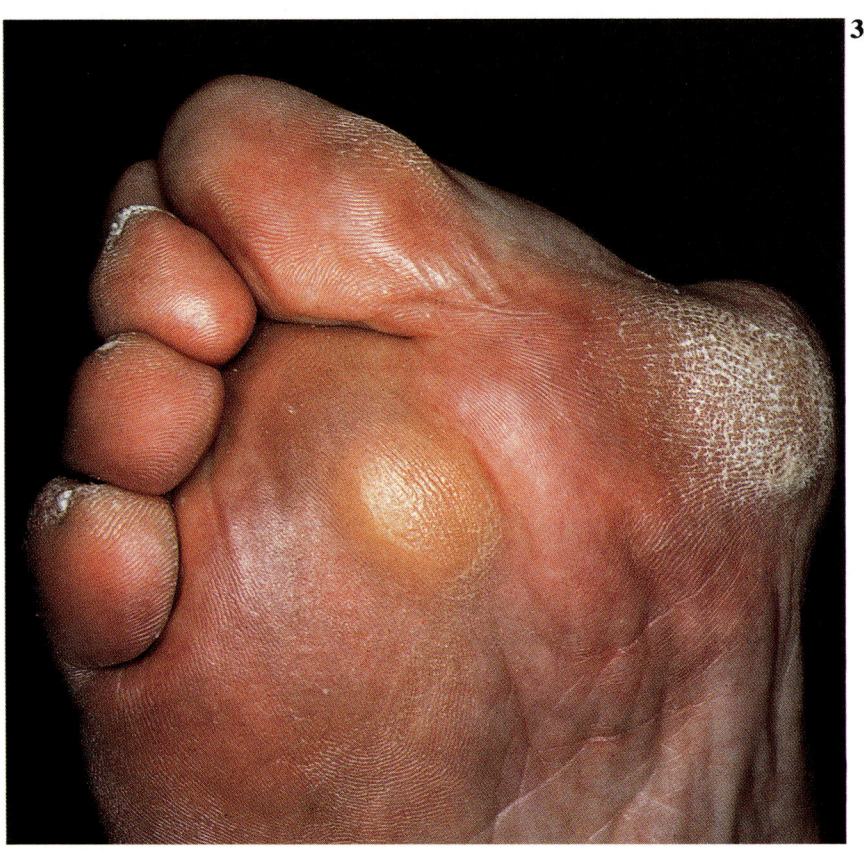

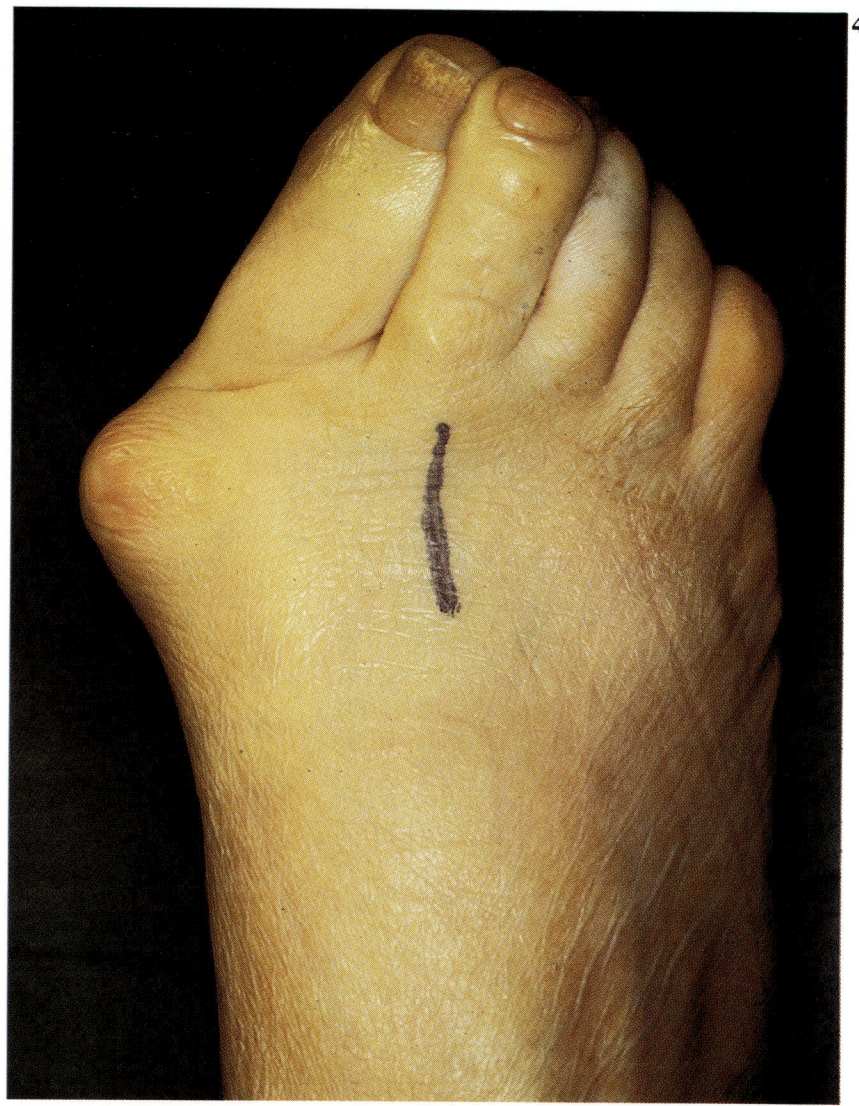

39 The line of bone section and displacement in metatarsal osteotomy.

40 **A longitudinal incision, 2.5 cm long, is made over the distal half of the appropriate metatarsal shaft.** If adjacent metatarsal bones are to be divided, a single incision can be made between them.

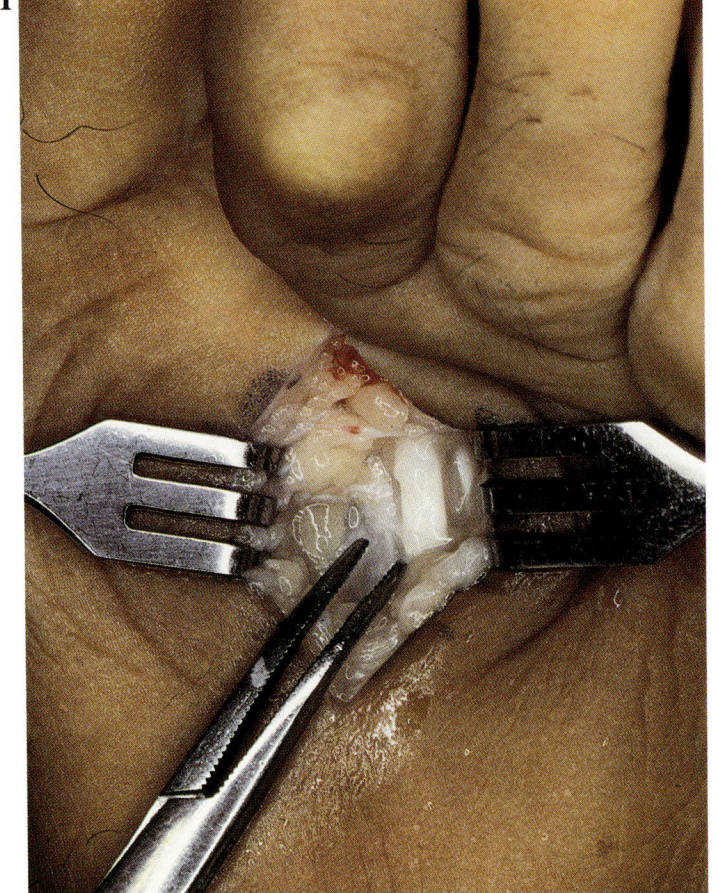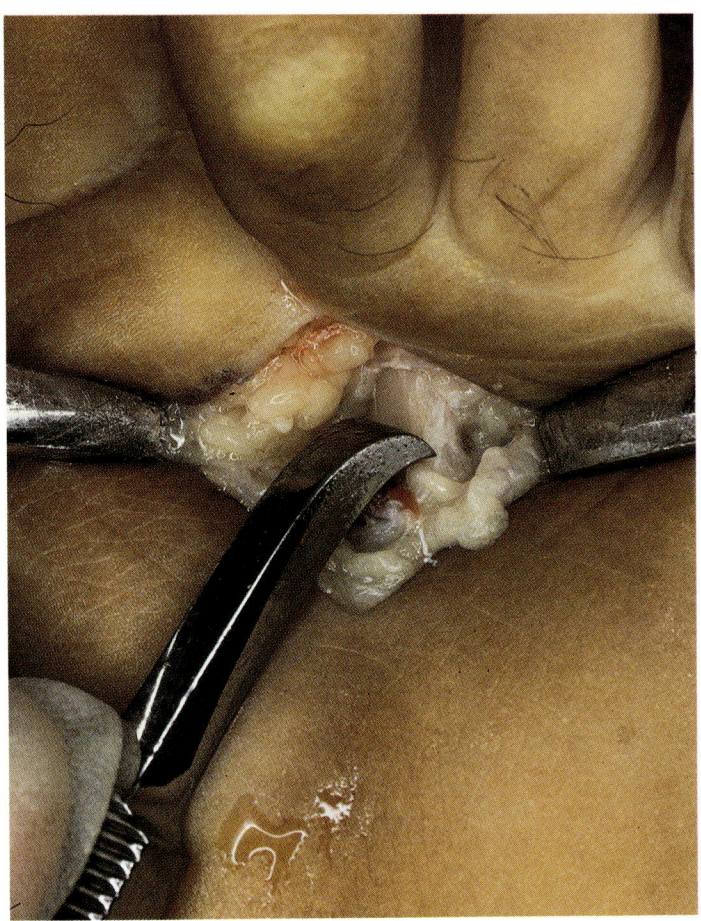

41 The incision is deepened, using blunt dissection. The extensor tendon is protected.

42 Using a small periosteal elevator, the metatarsal shaft is cleared.

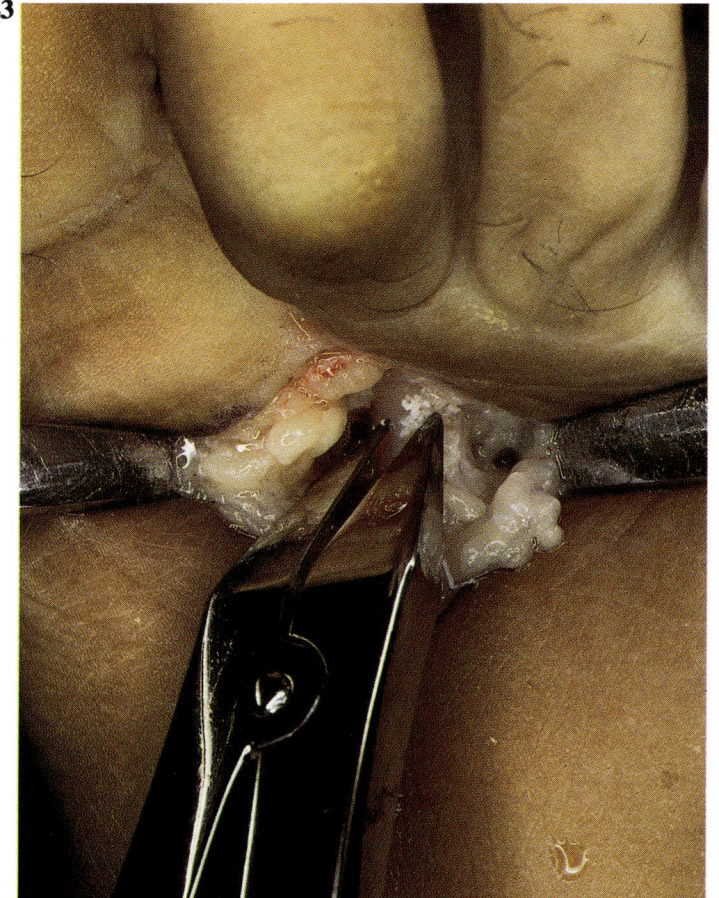

43 The bone is nibbled through using bone-cutting forceps. If it is cut through with one bite of the forceps, the bone may splinter. The osteotomy should slope 45 degrees downwards and distally.

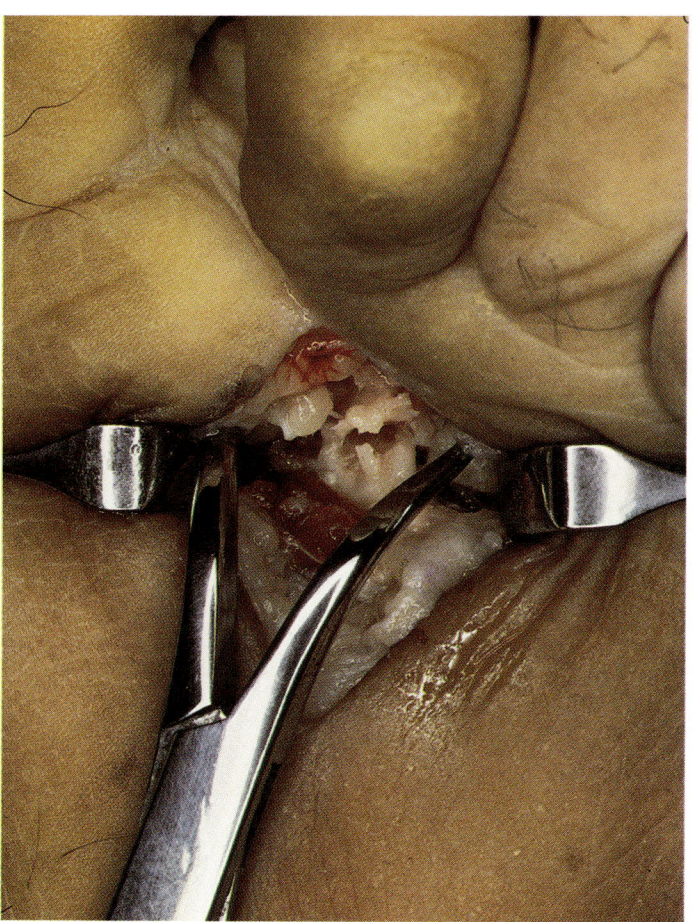

44 The metatarsal head is drawn proximally with bone-holding forceps, so that it slides up at the osteotomy site without angulating. Any prominent spike of bone on the distal fragment should be nibbled off. Skin is closed with interrupted 3–0 nylon sutures and the operation field is infiltrated with local anaesthetic (see **6**).

Postoperative management

A protective wool and crepe bandage is applied. Weight bearing is encouraged to ensure that the metatarsal head remains in its corrected position, but when the patient is not walking the foot should be kept elevated.

Complications

Specific complications are few. Fibrous union of the osteotomy has been reported but does not seem to cause problems. Stiffness of the metatarsophalangeal joints can be minimised by keeping the dissection well away from the joints and encouraging early mobilisation of the toes. If metatarsal osteotomy is combined with other operations that require postoperative plaster immobilisation, it is important to mould the sole of the plaster to retain the metatarsal head in the corrected position.

Hallux valgus — Keller's arthroplasty

This operation is indicated for the treatment of symptoms caused by severe hallux valgus in the elderly. Careful selection of patients is necessary; a desire to improve the appearance of the foot is not an indication for Keller's arthroplasty, and it should not be used to correct a hallux valgus deformity in young, active people. Correction of a hallux valgus deformity will not relieve metatarsalgia (see page **30**).

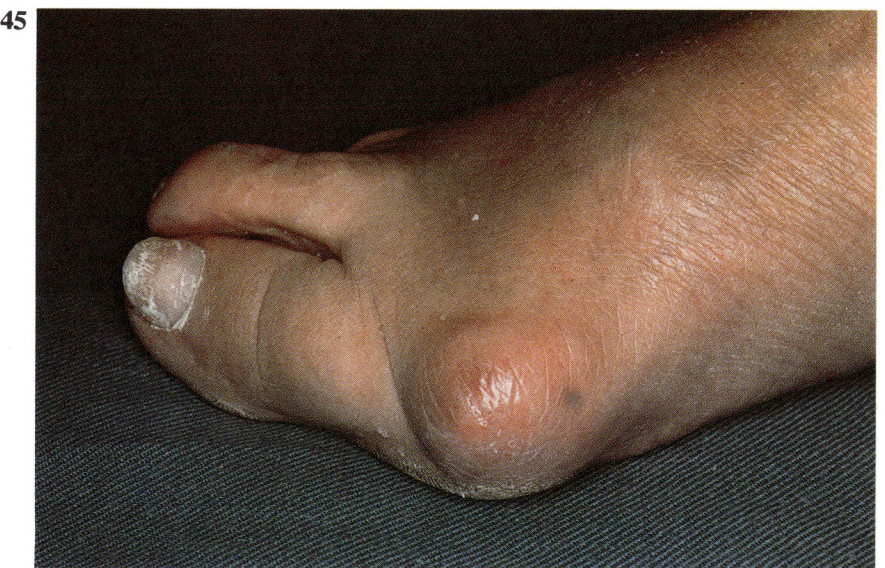

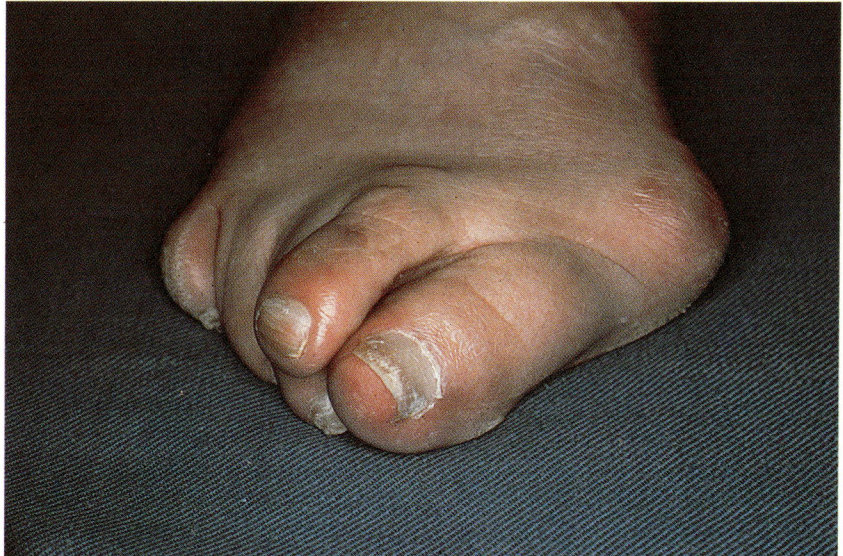

45 and 46 Hallux valgus. This patient had repeated infections in the bursa over the first metatarsal head and pain from shoe pressure on the bursa and callosities on the great toe. The second toe overrides the great toe and is subject to pressure from the front of the shoe.

The aim of the operation is to remove the medial eminence of the metatarsal head (often referred to as the 'exostosis', although it is not a true exostosis) and to realign the great toe by removing part of the proximal phalanx thus making the toe floppy.

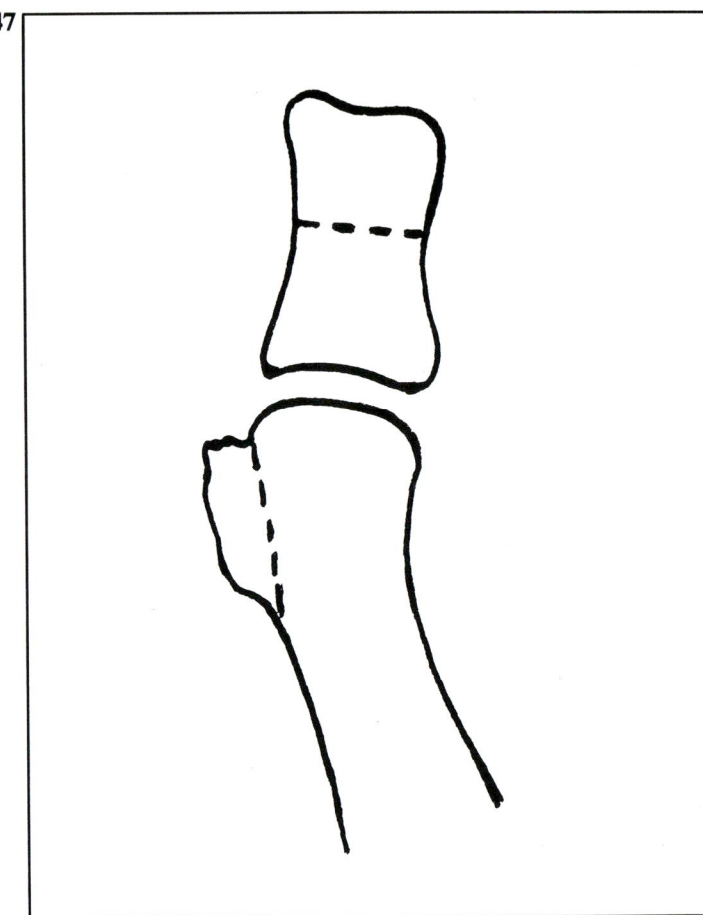

47 Bone resection in Keller's operation.

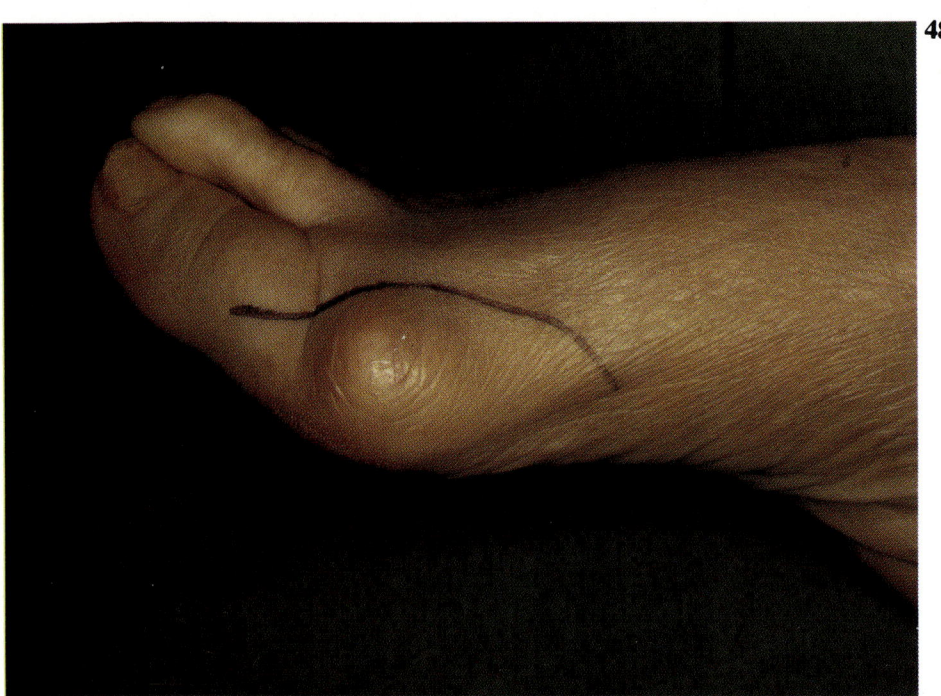

48 A curved incision extends from the proximal phalanx to the metatarsal neck.

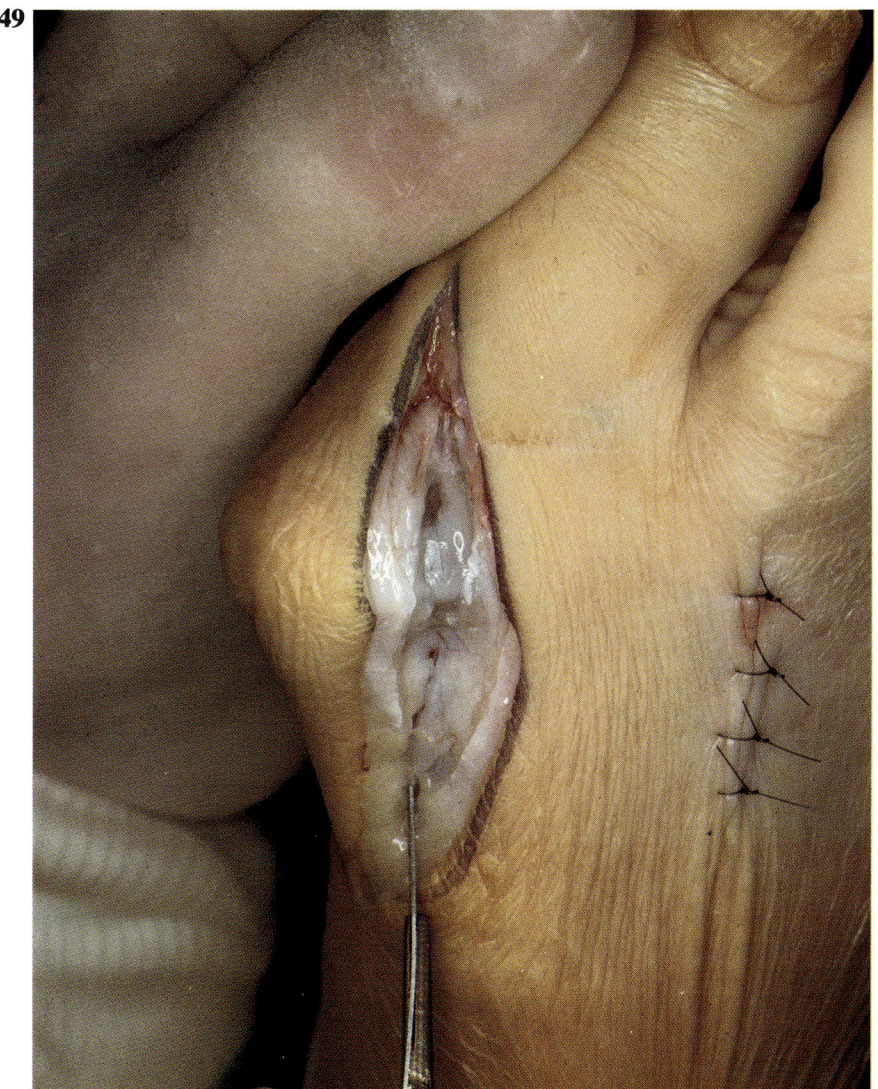

49 The incision is deepened to the bone. Small veins are coagulated and damage to the terminal branches of sensory nerves is avoided. (This patient has had an osteotomy of the second metatarsal bone.)

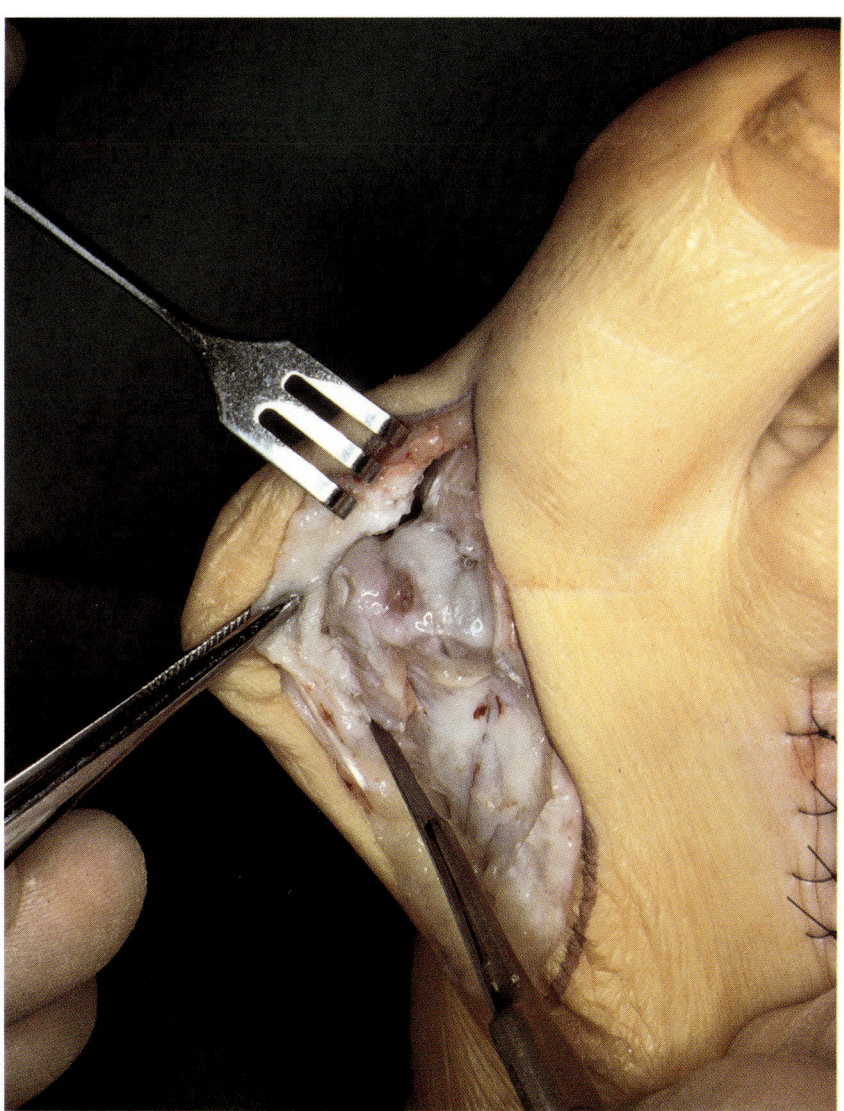

50 The skin and bursa on the medial aspect of the metatarsal head are raised by sharp dissection close to bone.

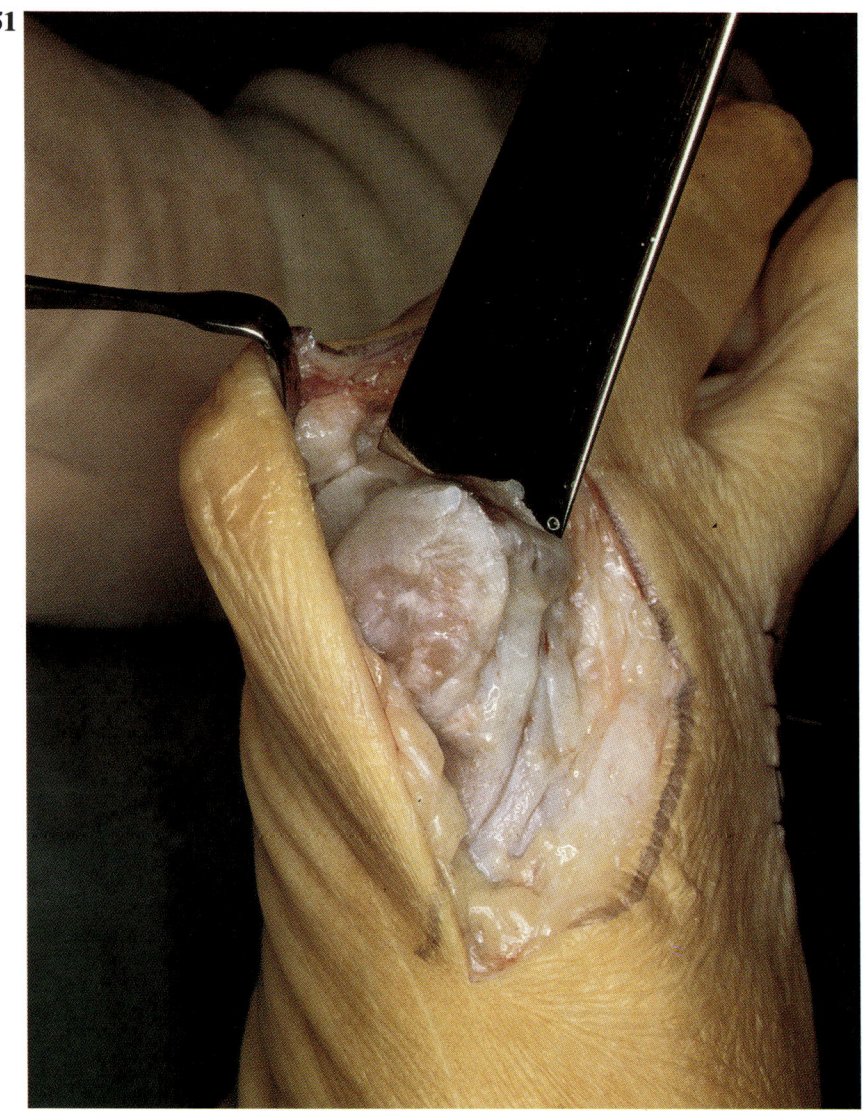
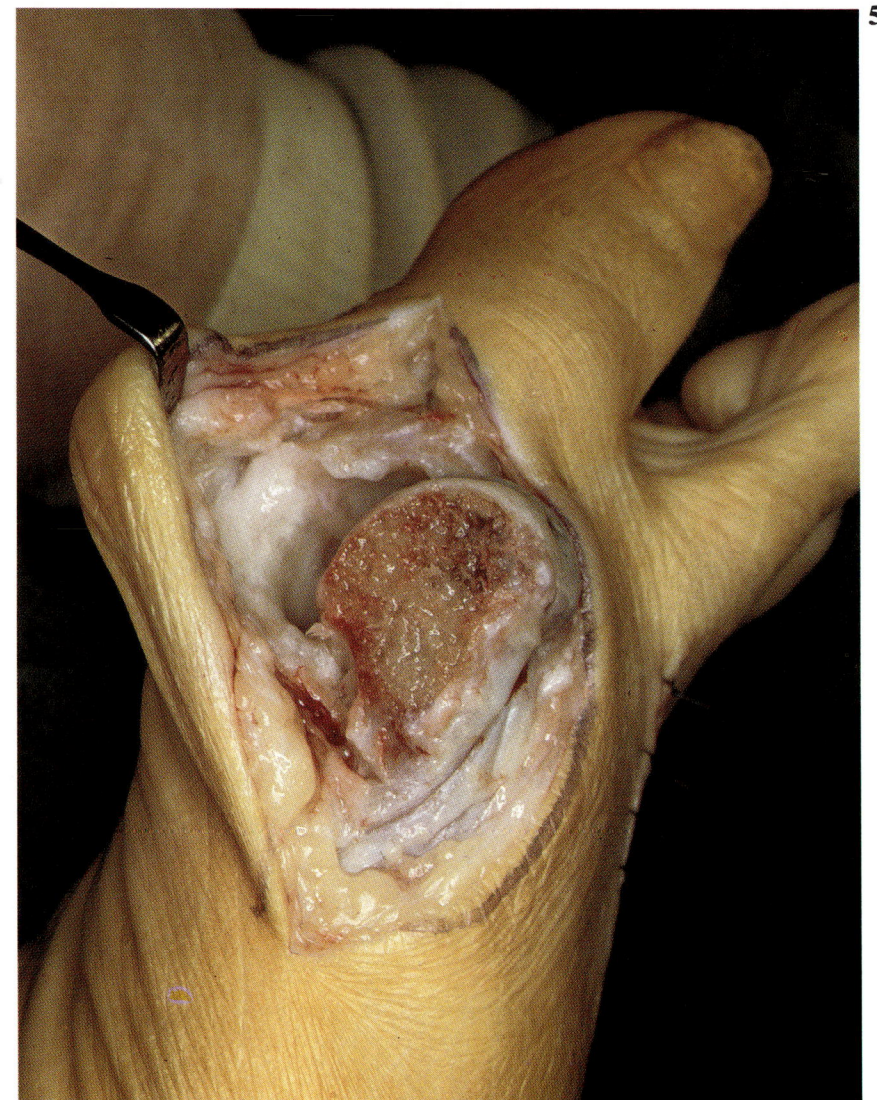

51 and 52　The 'exostosis' is trimmed off, flush with the metatarsal shaft, using an osteotome. Damage to the weight-bearing part of the metatarsal head must be avoided.

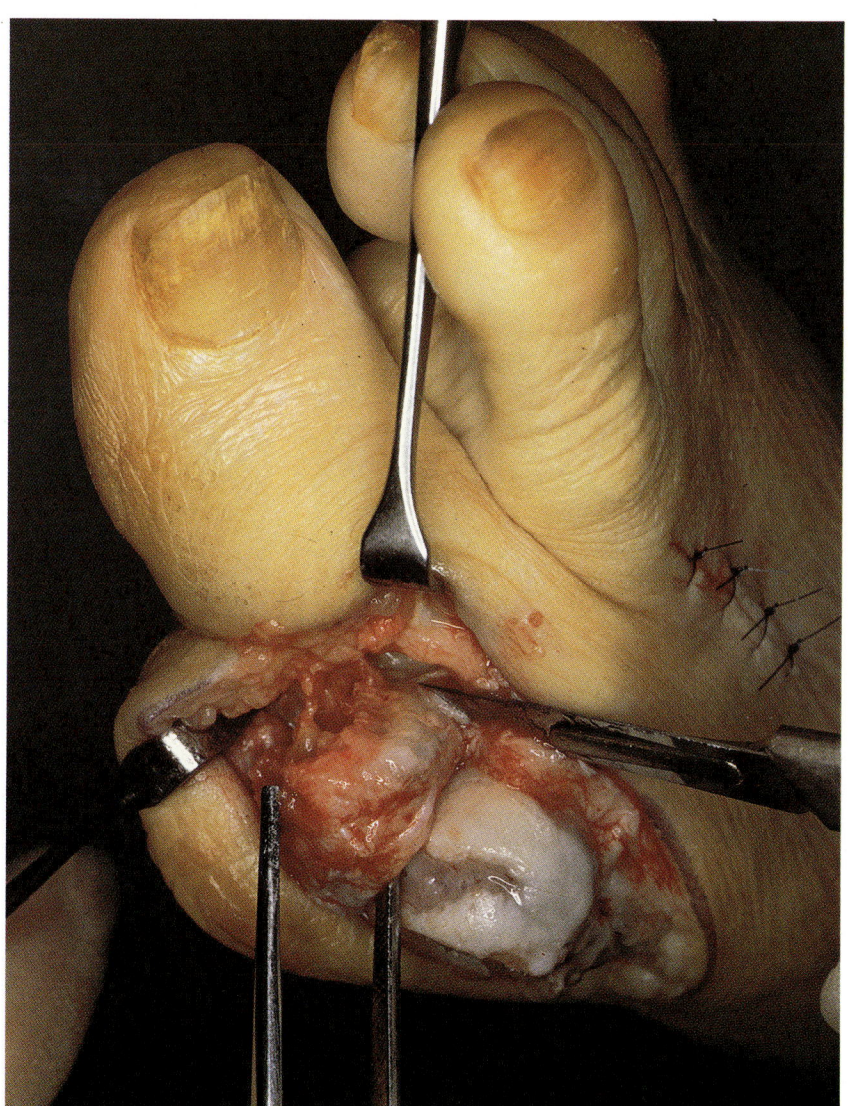

53 At least half of the proximal phalanx is removed by nibbling through the bone with pointed cutting forceps. A single bite of the forceps is avoided because of the risk of splintering the bone.

54 The fragment of bone is removed with its covering of periosteum.

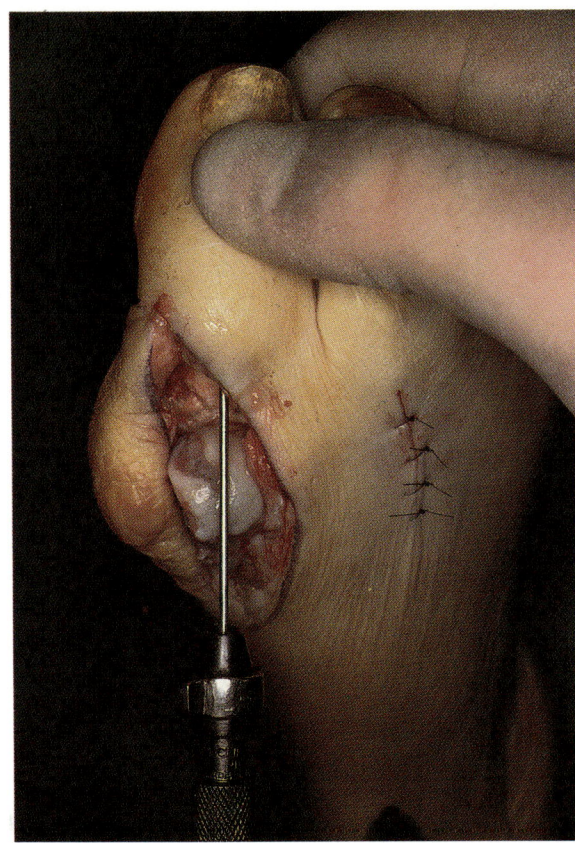

55 A 0.062" diameter double-ended Kirschner wire is driven up the toe by hand or power drill. The drill is then transferred to the other end of the wire which is withdrawn completely into the toe.

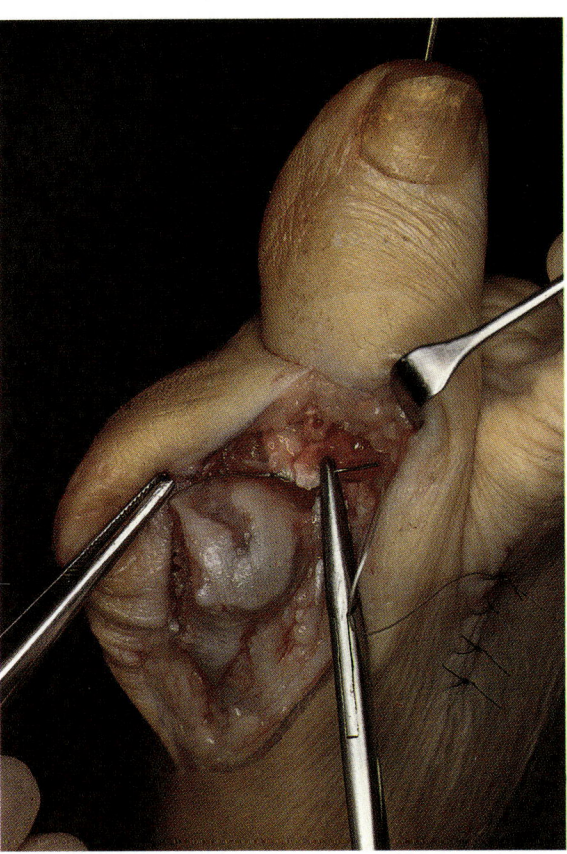

56 Loose soft tissue is drawn over the raw surface of the proximal phalanx with a purse-string suture of Dexon or Vicryl.

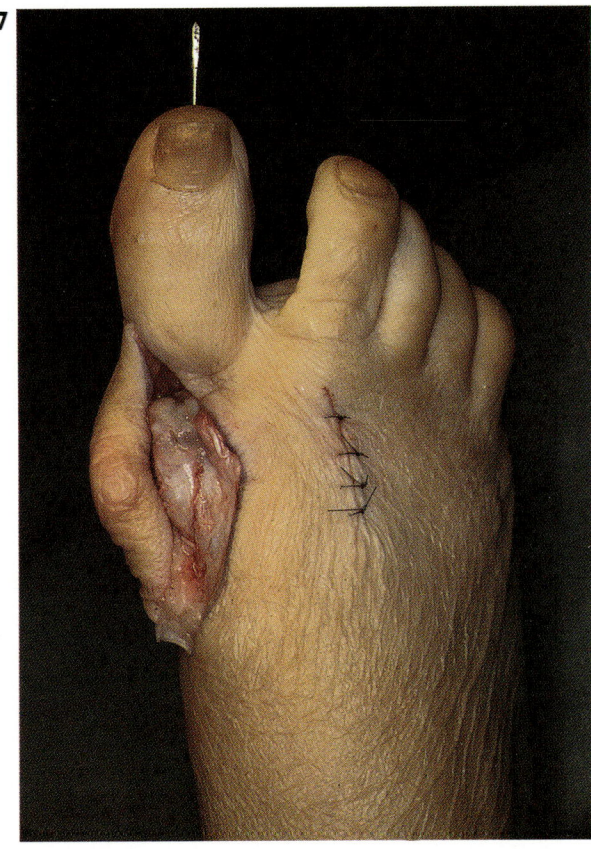

57 The K-wire is then driven into the metatarsal bone and should maintain a gap of at least 1 cm between the metatarsal head and the proximal phalanx. If the tendon of extensor hallucis longus is tight, it should be lengthened with a Z-cut and resutured.

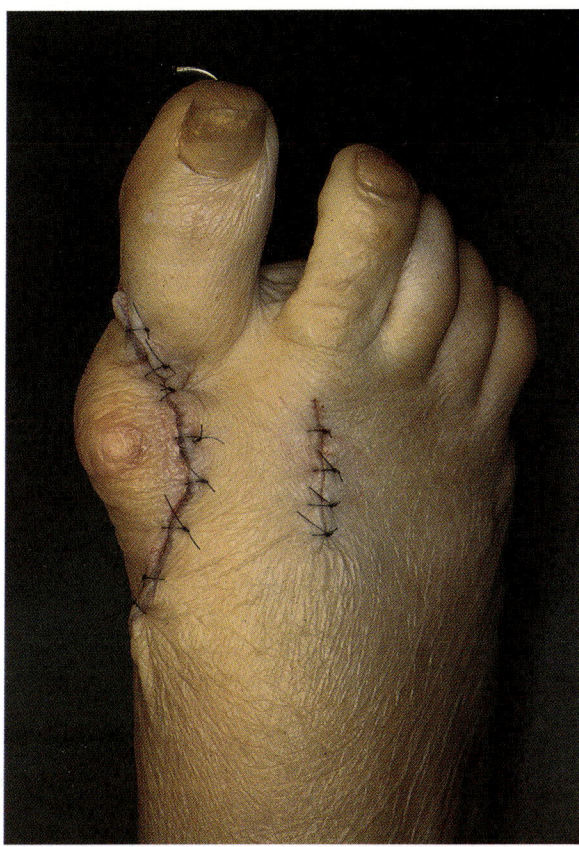

58 Final appearance. After confirming that the K-wire has a good grip in the metatarsal bone (see **23**), the wire is cut short and bent over. Skin is closed with interrupted 3–0 nylon sutures. Bupivacaine is infiltrated into the wound.

Postoperative management

The foot is kept elevated as much as possible to minimise swelling, but a limited amount of walking may be allowed in a protective plaster toe splint which is worn for three weeks after operation, until the sutures and the K-wire are removed. Thereafter walking is gradually increased. Many patients find that a firm-soled shoe with a cut-out over the toes provides suitable footwear at this stage. Normal footwear can be worn about 6 to 8 weeks after operation; a simple block splint between the toes will help maintain correction.

Complications

Early complications after Keller's arthroplasty are similar to those that may occur after arthrodesis of the first metatarsophalangeal joint (page **23**) and are prevented or dealt with in the same way.

Hallux valgus — Mitchell's osteotomy

In young, active people who have symptoms caused by a hallux valgus deformity first metatarsal osteotomy is preferable to Keller's operation. Mitchell's osteotomy shifts the metatarsal head laterally and proximally, correcting the bony deformity and relaxing the soft tissues that contribute a deforming force on the toe. This operation requires precise technique and a powered bone saw is essential. This procedure is contraindicated if there are degenerative changes in the metatarsophalangeal joint of the great toe.

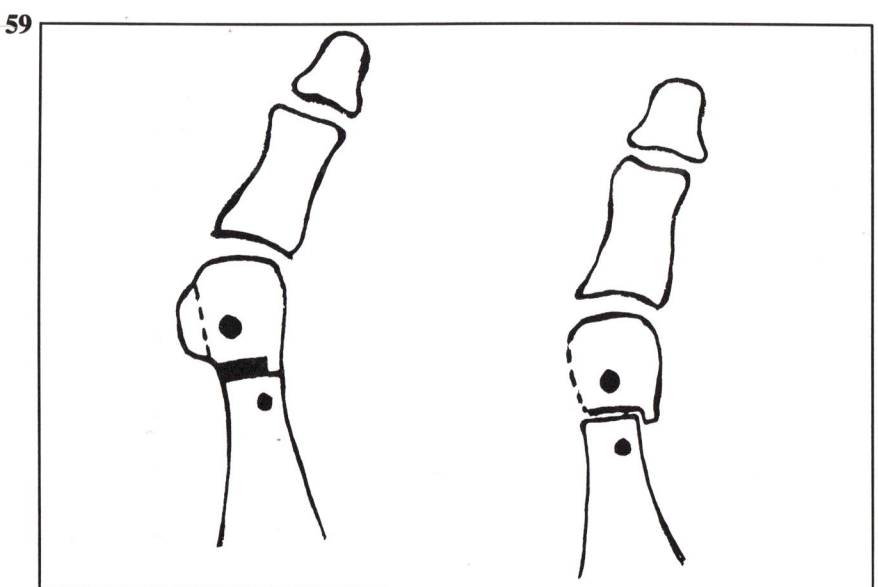

59 Mitchell's osteotomy.

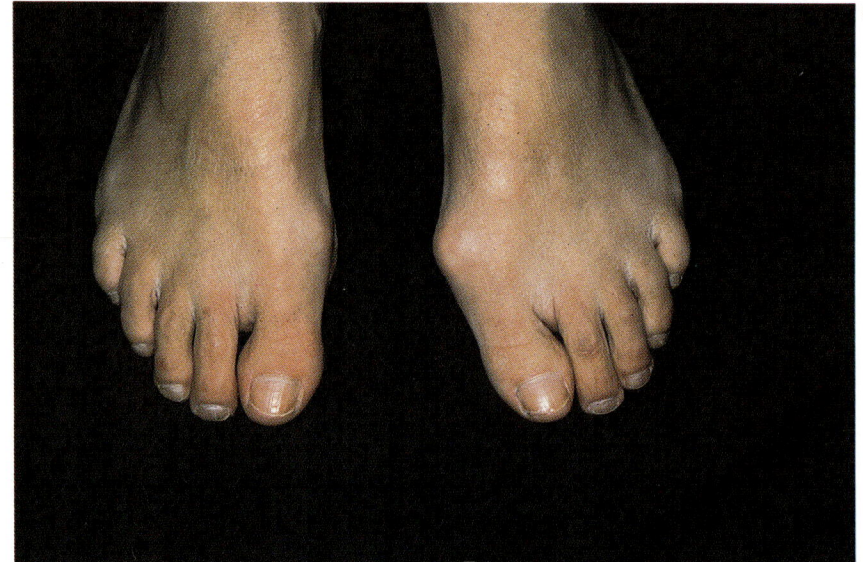

60 Left hallux valgus in a 24-year-old woman. She complained of discomfort and recurrent infection in the region of the medial prominence of the metatarsal head. She also complained that she had difficulty obtaining satisfactory shoes.

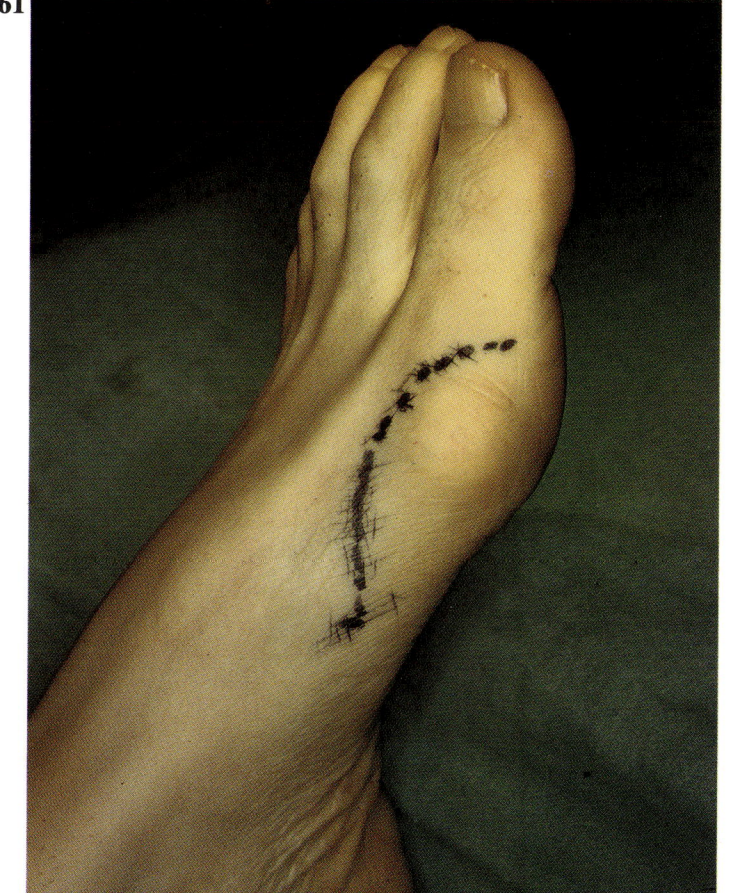

61 The incision curves dorsally over the 'exostosis'.

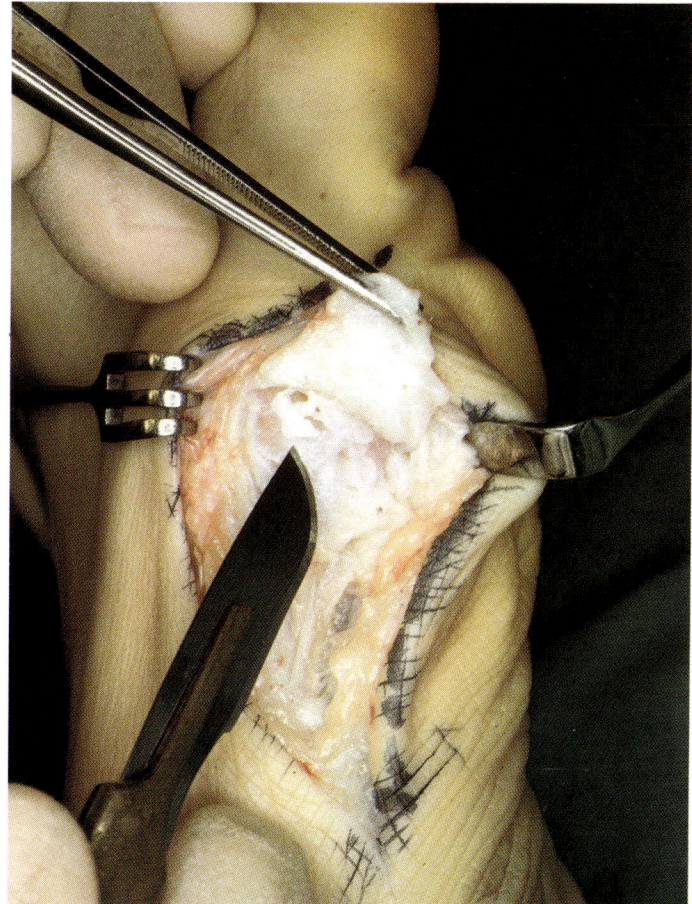

62 Care is taken not to open the metatarsophalangeal joint. Small veins are coagulated with diathermy. The soft tissue over the medial prominence of the metatarsal head is raised as a triangular flap with a distal base.

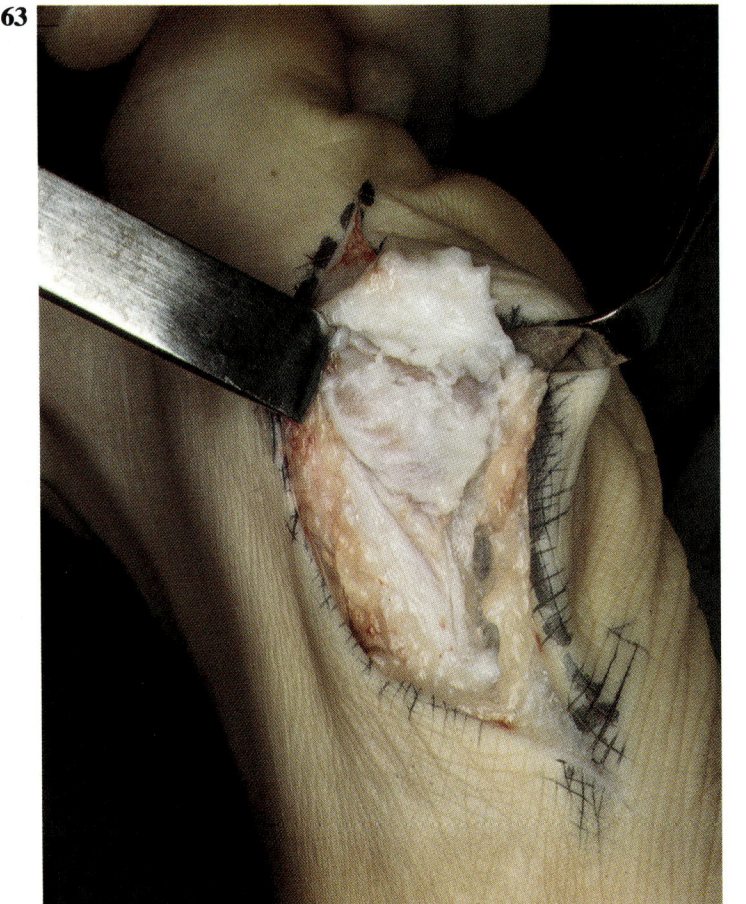
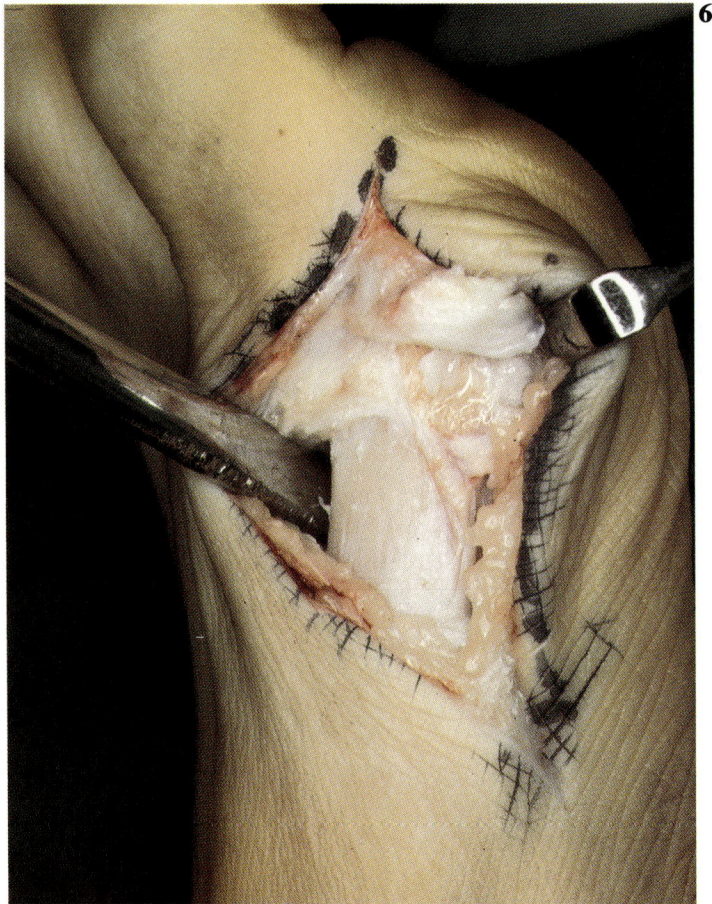

63 The 'exostosis' is removed with an osteotome.

64 Periosteum is elevated from the metatarsal neck.

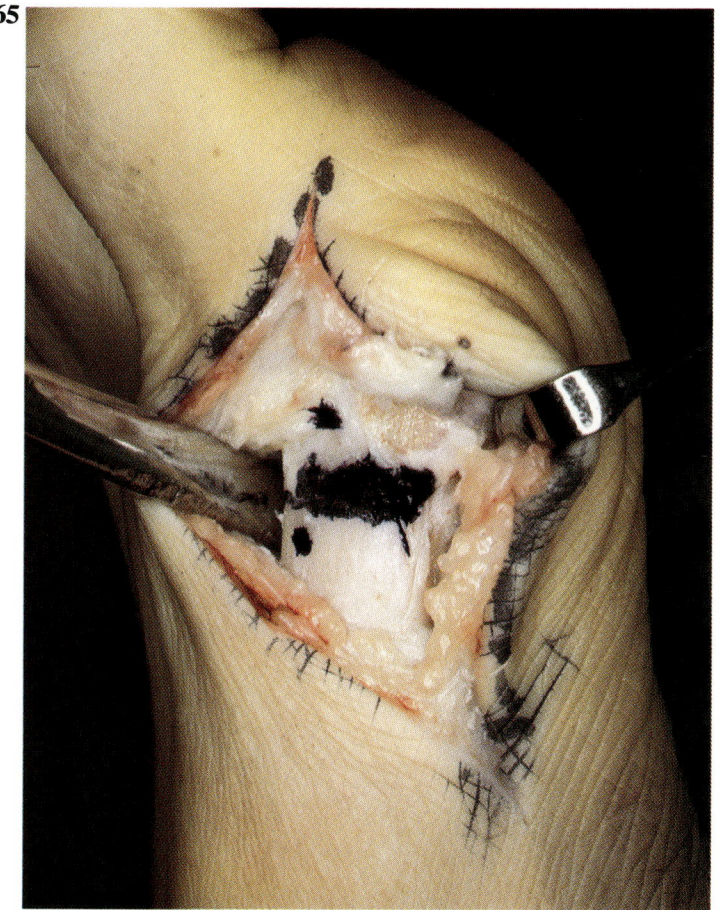
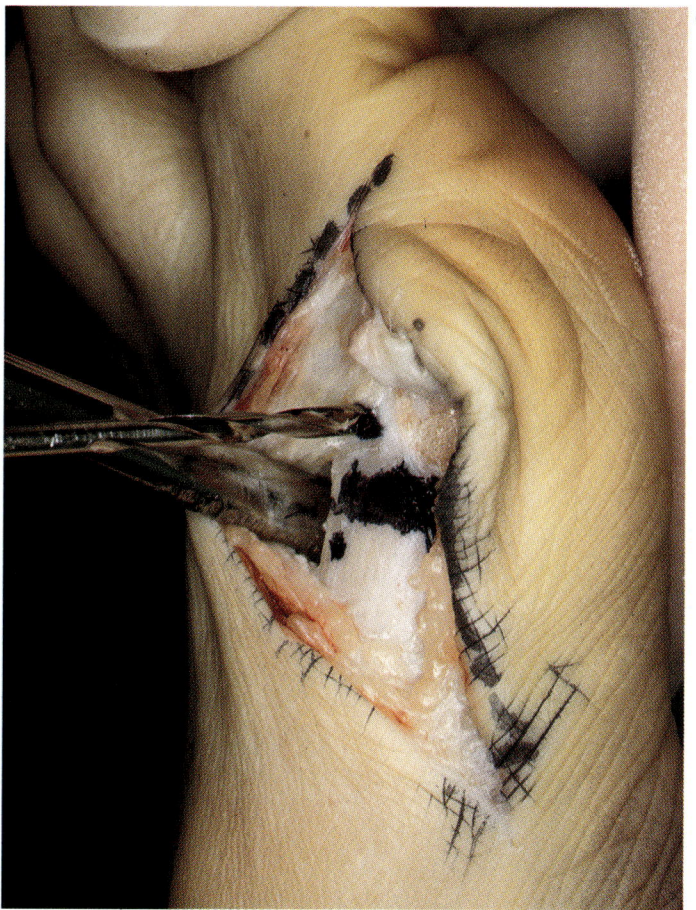

65 The drill holes and the line of the osteotomy have been indicated with surgical marking ink. The level of the osteotomy is about 1.5 cm from the joint, just proximal to the medial prominence of the metatarsal head. A slice of bone about 2 mm thick will be removed.

66 The two holes are drilled vertically towards the sole using a 2 mm drill. Each hole lies at least 0.5 cm from the line of the osteotomy; the two holes are parallel but offset (see **59**).

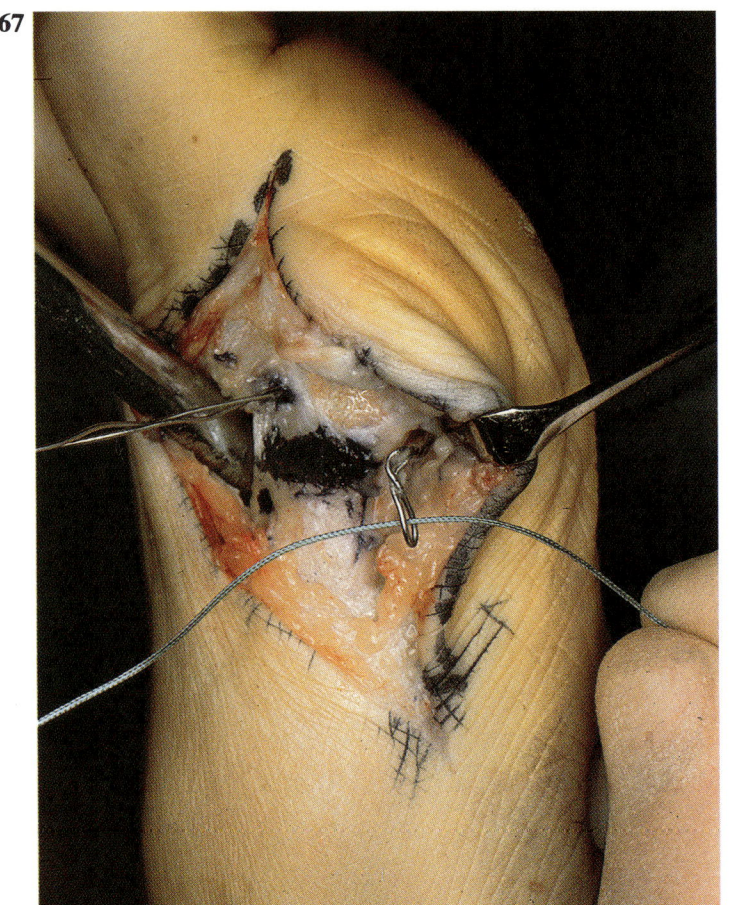

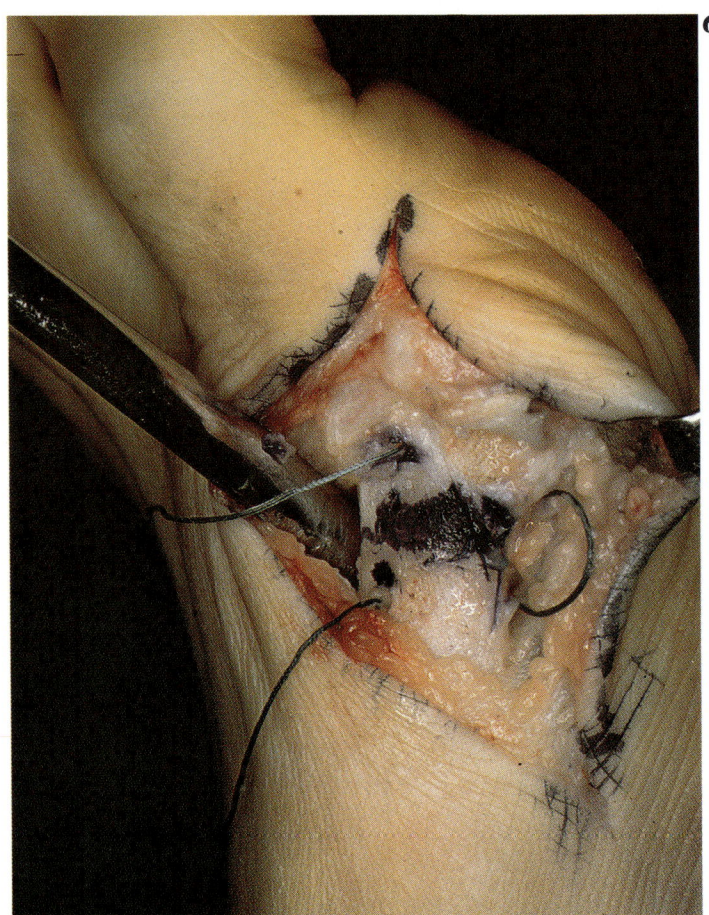

67 A loop of 20 swg wire, twisted to form an eye, is passed through one of the drill holes in a plantar direction. The end of a length of stout absorbable suture (such as O Dexon) is passed through the eye and the loop withdrawn.

68 The procedure is repeated, passing the wire through the other hole and withdrawing the other end of the suture.

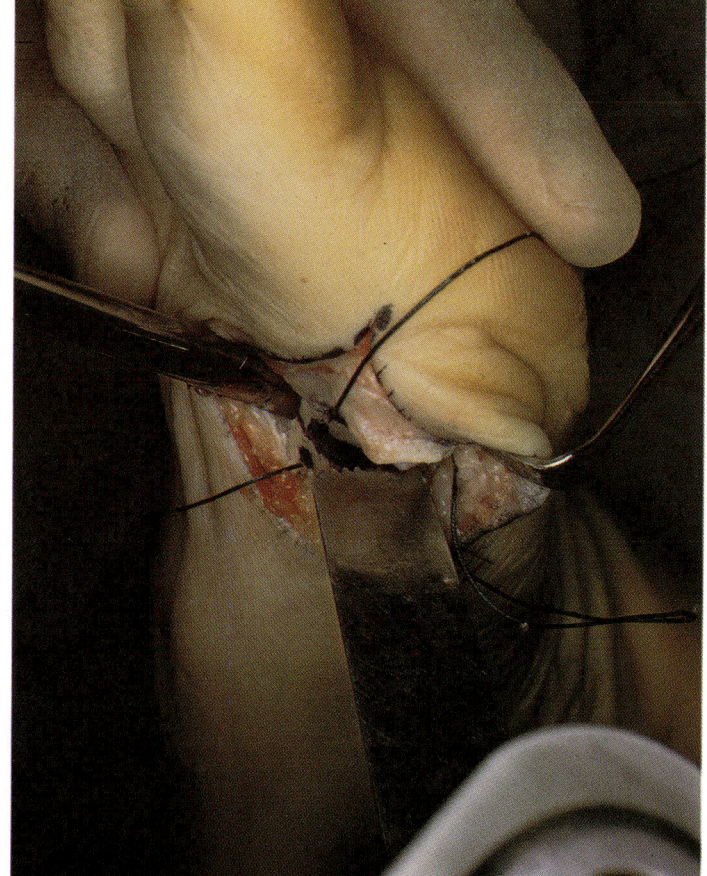
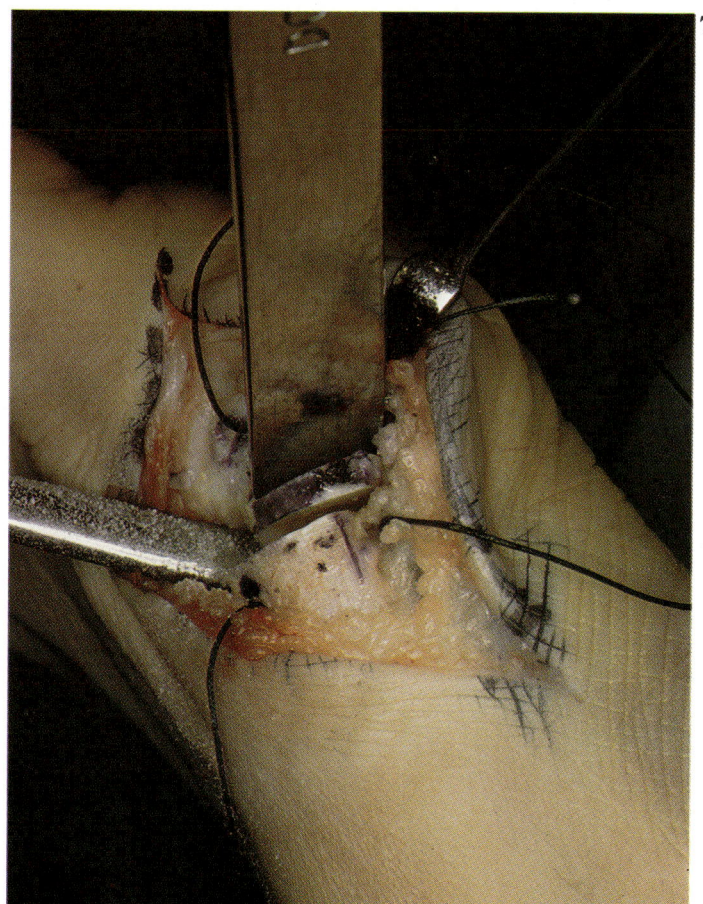

69 **A powered saw is used to make the osteotomy.** The distal cut is made first and extends about 80 per cent across the metatarsal bone. The proximal cut extends right across. The cuts should converge very slightly in the plantar direction to bring the metatarsal head into a slightly plantarflexed position. Dorsiflexion of the metatarsal head must be avoided, to prevent excessive weight being thrown onto the second metatarsal head.

70 **The osteotomy is opened and the slice of bone is removed by levering it off with an osteotome.**

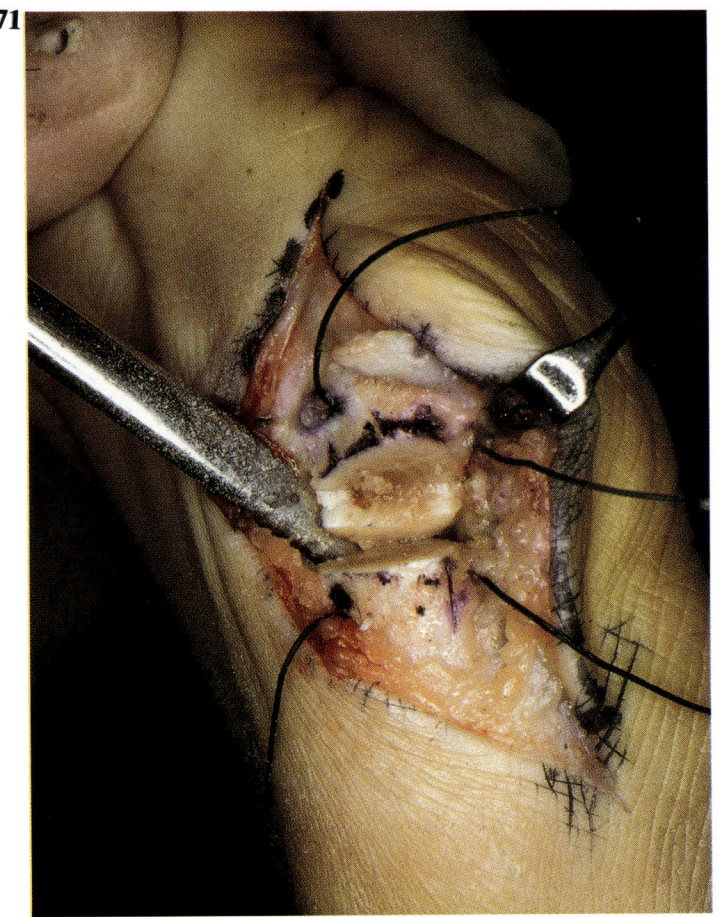 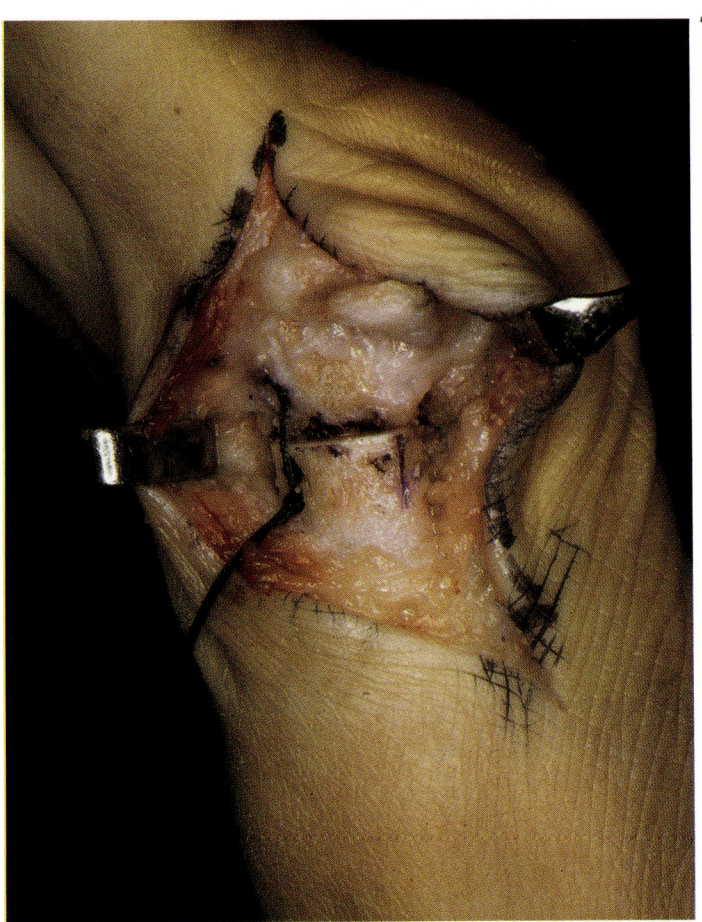

71 The amount of displacement of the metatarsal head is dictated by the width of the piece of bone left attached to it; if the displacement is too much, a little more bone should be removed.

72 When the position is judged to be satisfactory the interosseous suture is tied tightly.

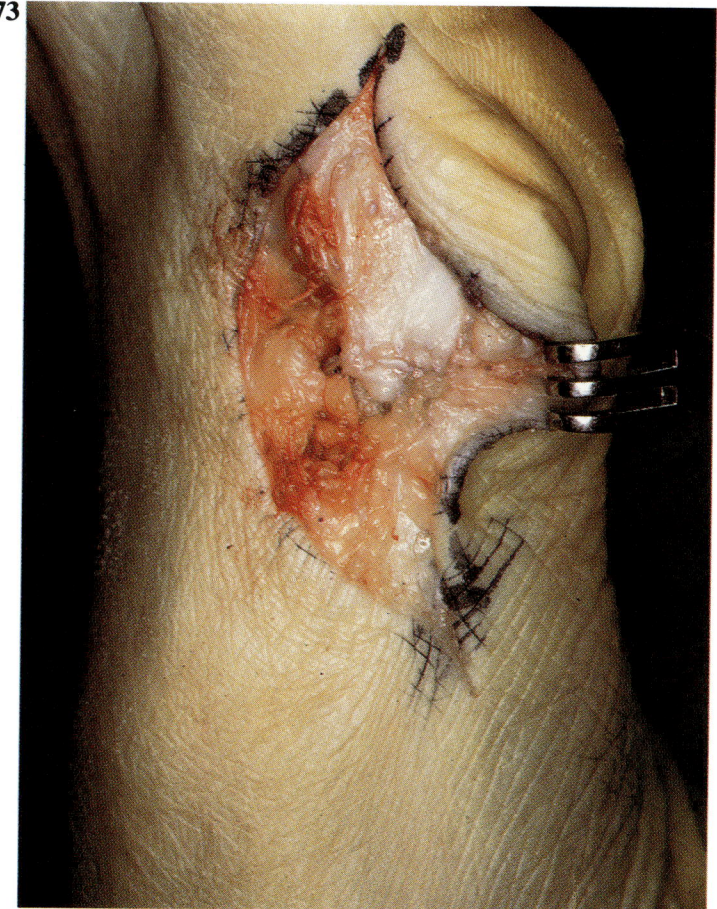 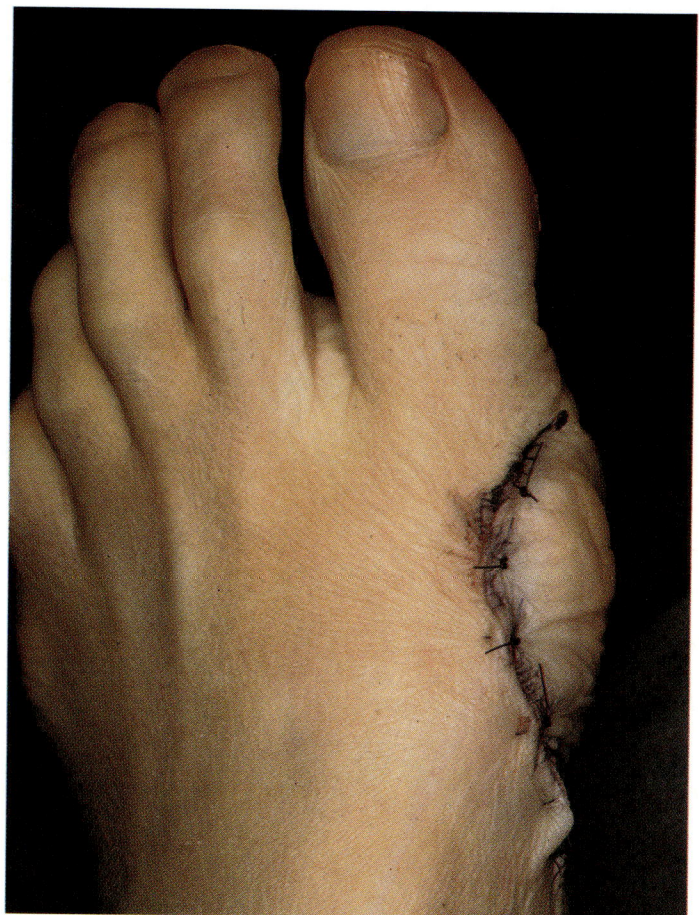

73 The interosseous suture holds the osteotomy in place, while the flap of soft tissue is drawn back over the osteotomy site and held with absorbable (Dexon or Vicryl) sutures. Displacement of the osteotomy is then unlikely, and more rigid stabilisation with a Kirschner wire or interosseous wire suture is unnecessary.

74 Skin is closed with interrupted 3–0 nylon sutures and the wound is infiltrated with 0.5 per cent bupivacaine, as usual.

Postoperative management

A wool and crepe bandage is applied and the foot is kept elevated for a few days. The foot is then placed in a below-knee non-weight-bearing plaster with a protective toe extension. A walking heel is added when the sutures are removed two weeks after operation. The plaster is retained for six weeks in all. Check radiograph are taken postoperatively and on removal of the plaster.

Complications

Complications are very few if the operation is performed carefully with attention to all the details mentioned above. Swelling and infection are dealt with along the lines described previously, should they occur. As noted, dorsiflexion of the metatarsal head should be avoided, because it may cause metatarsalgia under the second metatarsal head. Avascular necrosis of the first metatarsal head can be a complication of excessive stripping of soft tissue from the lateral side of the neck of the metatarsal bone.

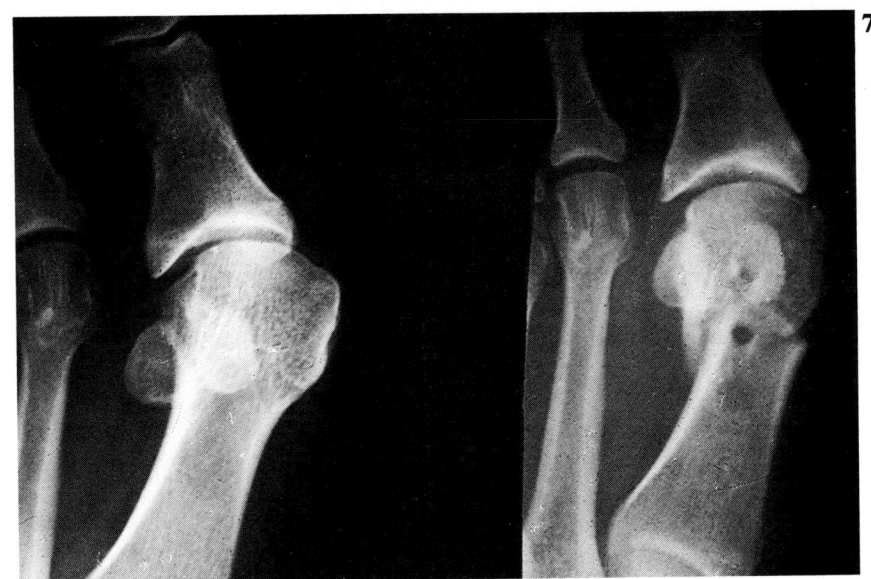

75 Radiographic appearances before and after operation.

Overriding fifth toe

This common congenital deformity does not correct spontaneously. However, the toe can be held in satisfactory alignment with a toe splint and this, combined with passive stretching of the toe into flexion and abduction, is the only treatment necessary in childhood. Surgical treatment is delayed until late childhood or adolescence. The usual reasons for operation are to relieve pressure on the toe from the shoe and to improve the appearance of the foot.

Several surgical procedures have been described for this condition; Butler's operation will be described.

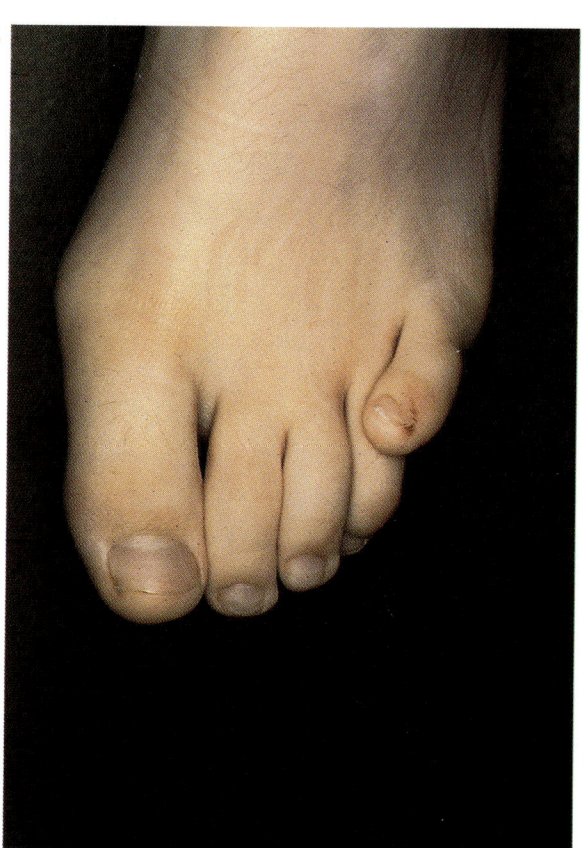

76 Overriding fifth toe in a girl aged 12 years.

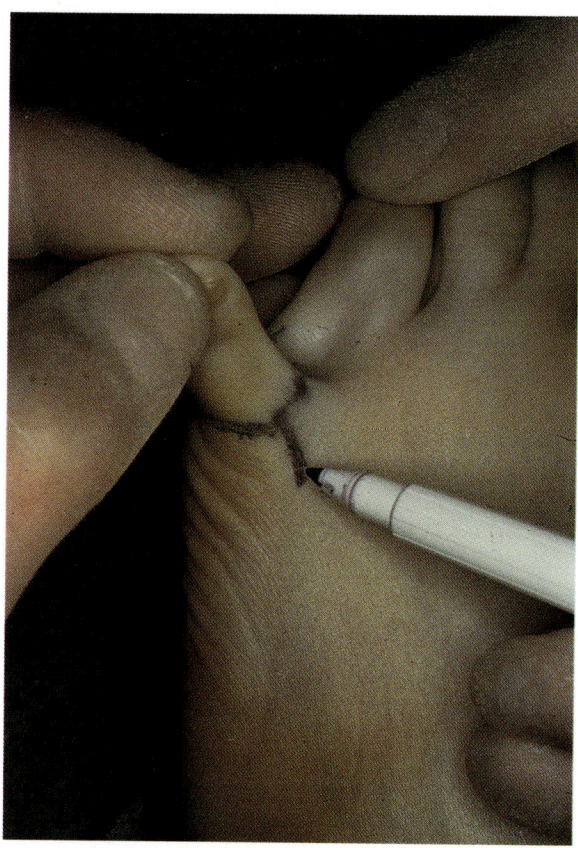

77 A racquet incision with a dorsal handle is marked out at the base of the toe.

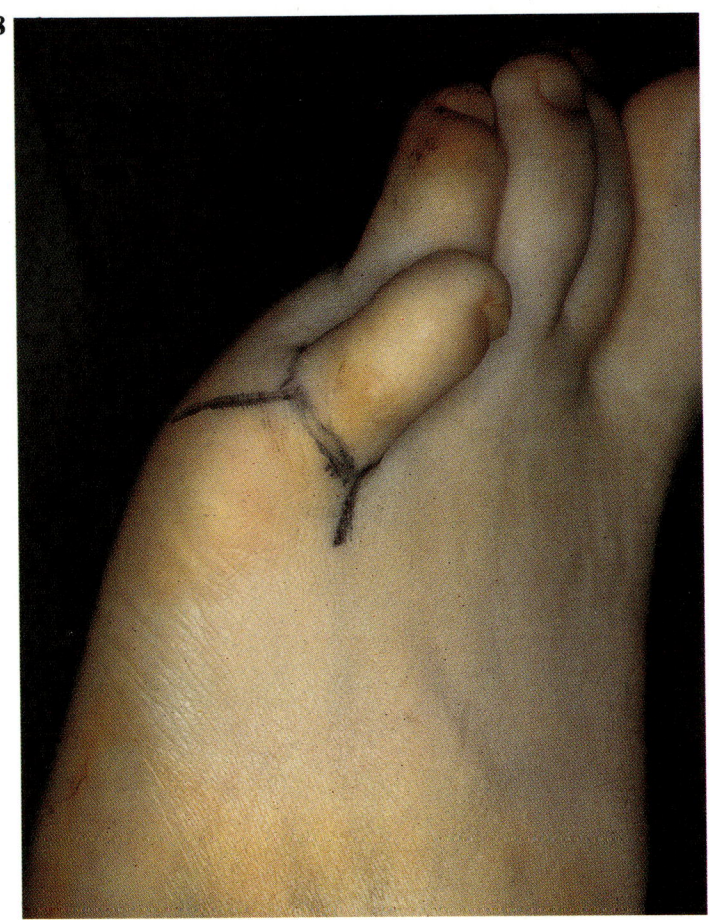

78 A second handle is added on the lateral border of the foot and extending to the plantar surface. The second racquet handle is slightly larger than the first.

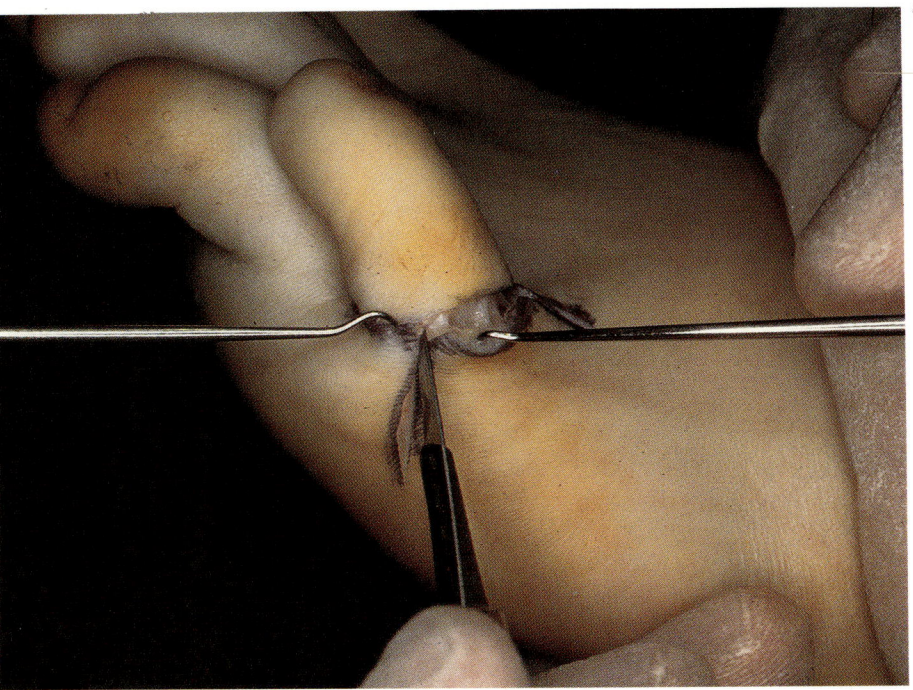

79 The flaps are raised proximally, being careful to keep the dissection in the subcutaneous plane.

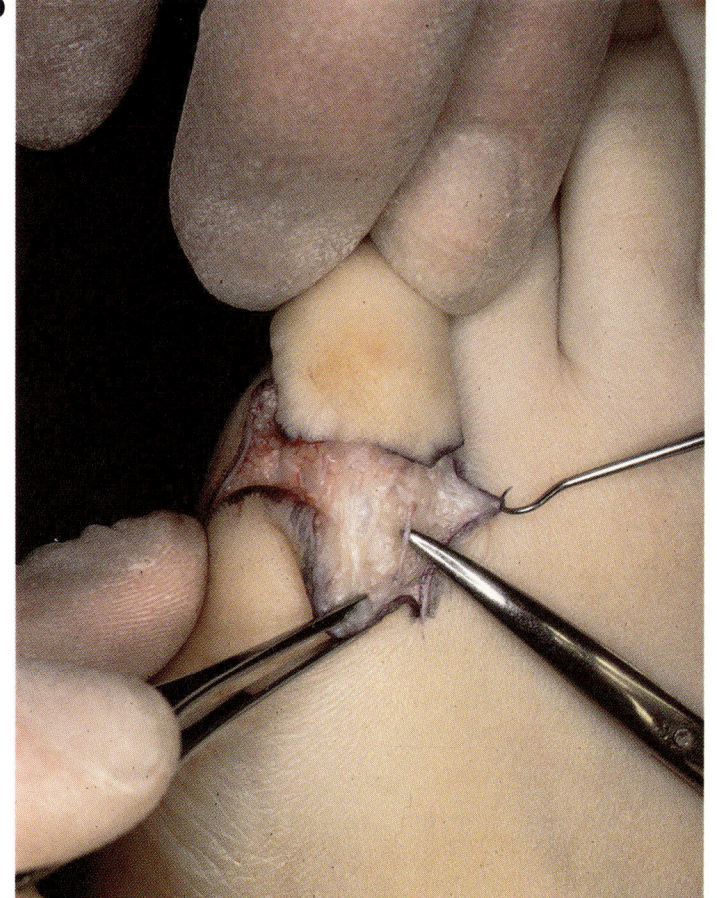

80 Dorsal veins are protected as are the plantar vessels and nerves. Damage to these structures is unlikely if the flaps are raised by blunt dissection.

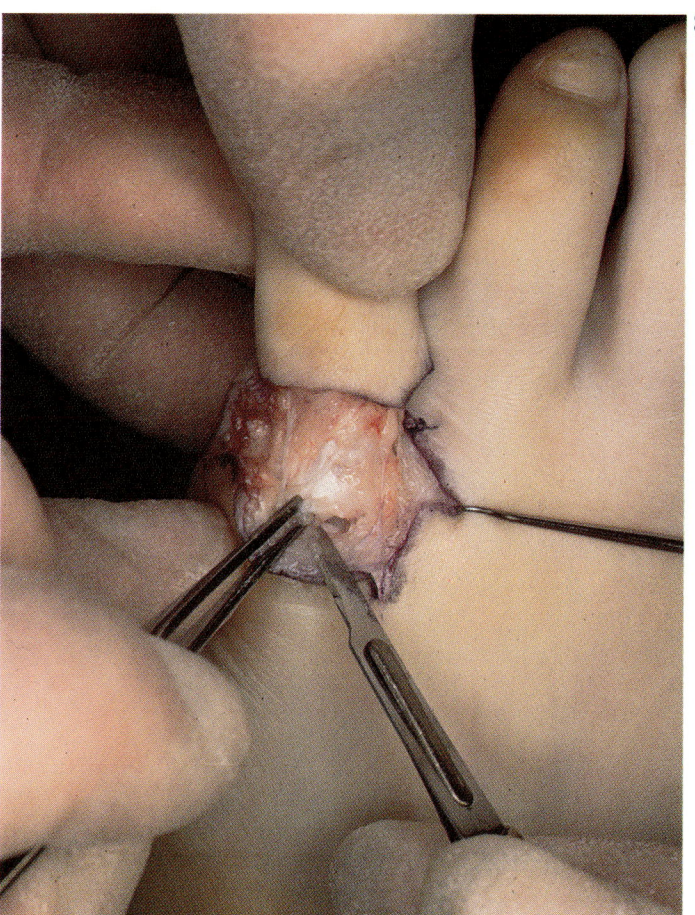

81 The extensor tendon and the dorsomedial capsule are divided with a knife.

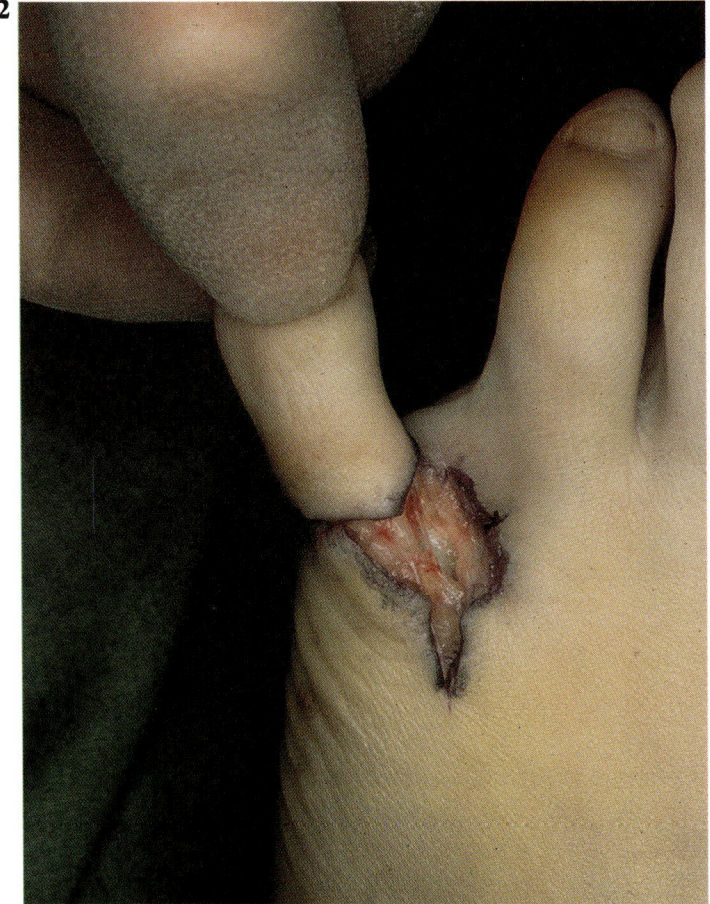

82 The toe can then be displaced into the plantar handle of the incision and can be abducted. It must lie in the corrected position without tension.

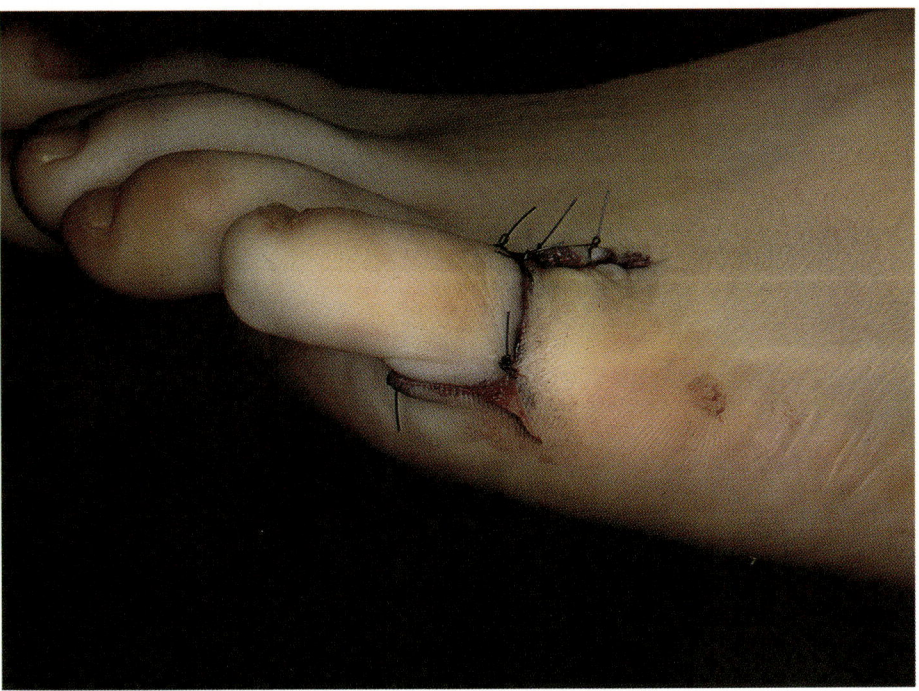

83 The toe is held in the corrected position by closing the skin with interrupted 4–0 nylon sutures. The plantar part of the incision is now much shorter. Local anaesthetic is instilled.

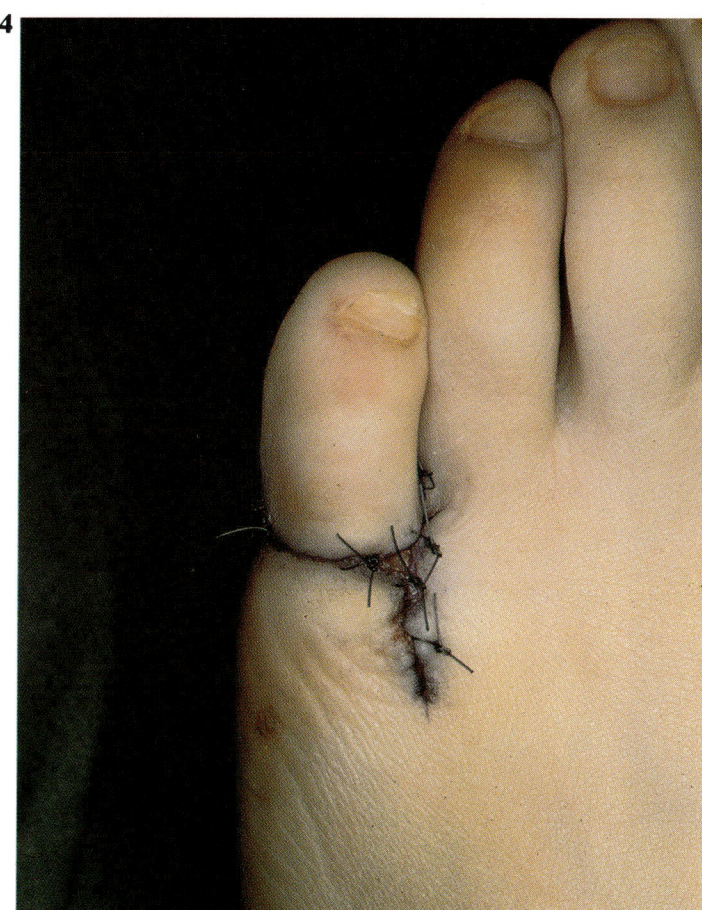

84　The corrected position.

Postoperative management

A light dressing is applied. Splintage is not necessary but, as usual, elevation of the foot is encouraged. Sutures are removed 10 to 14 days after operation; normal activity and footwear are then allowed.

Complications

Specific complications are uncommon. There may be a risk of endangering the circulation if the toe is very contracted; for this reason the operation is not recommended in adults.

Plantar digital neuroma

In this condition (also known as Morton's neuroma) there is fibrosis and enlargement of the branch of the medial plantar nerve lying between the third and fourth metatarsal heads. The pathogenesis is obscure, and the lesion is certainly not a true neuroma, but the clinical picture is characteristic. The middle-aged are most frequently affected; the typical sufferer experiences sudden episodes of severe neuralgic pain shooting into the third and fourth toes when walking. Pain is sometimes eased by removing the shoe and massaging the affected area. The diagnosis is made from the typical history; clinical examination is often negative but pressure over the neuroma or pressing the two metatarsal heads together may elicit the same discomfort. Immediate relief of symptoms is obtained by resection of the affected nerve.

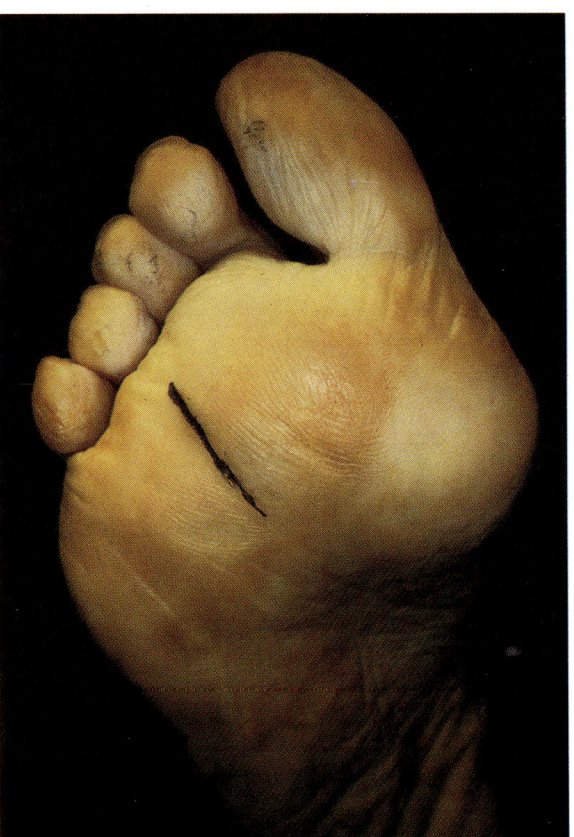

85 A longitudinal plantar incision about 3 cm long between the third and fourth metatarsal heads is preferred. A dorsal approach is not recommended, because it can be difficult to resect the nerve sufficiently proximal when this approach is used.

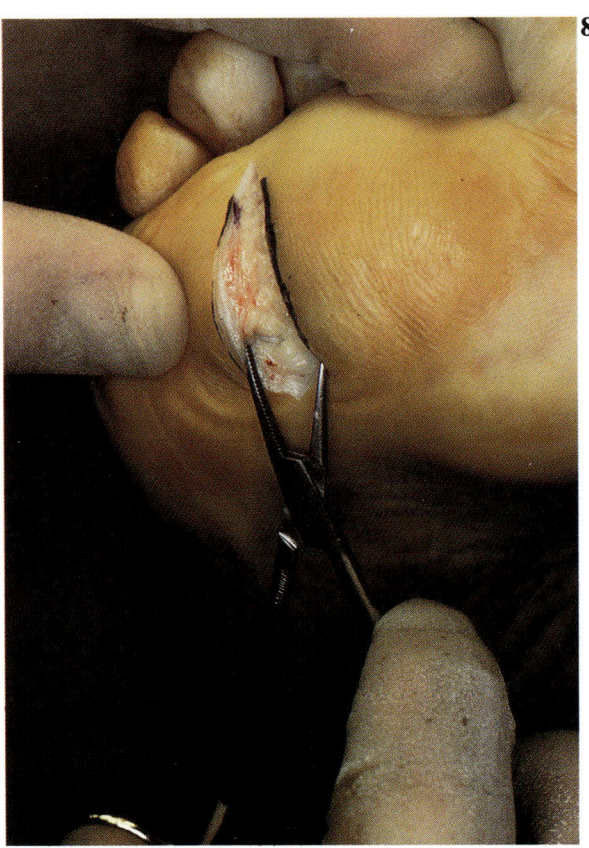

86 The incision is deepened down to the metatarsal heads by blunt dissection.

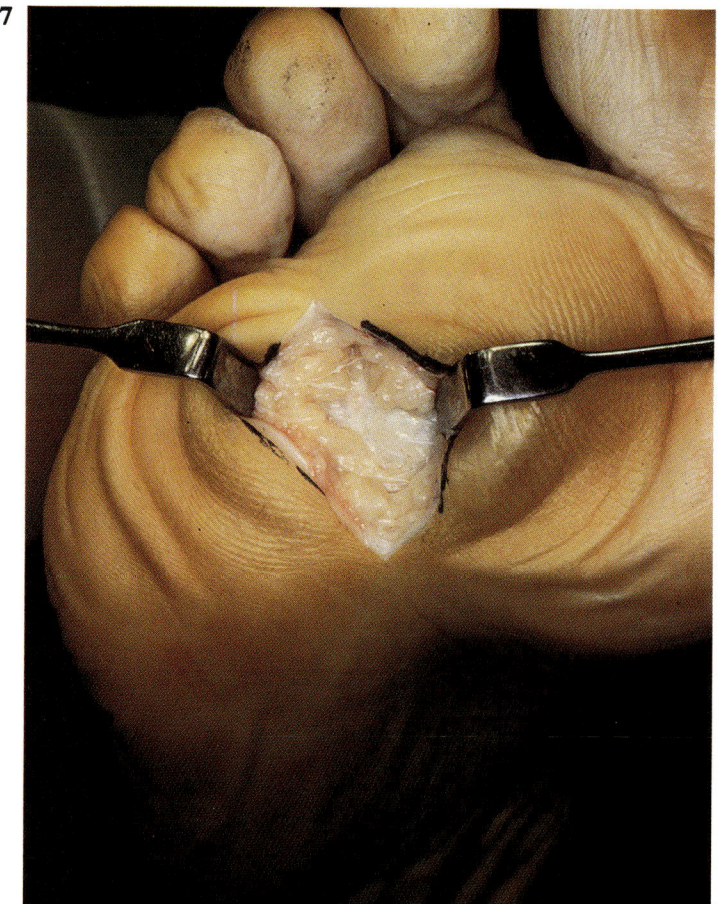

87 Fat bulges into the wound. It can be trimmed back with scissors and held out of the way with a self-retaining retractor.

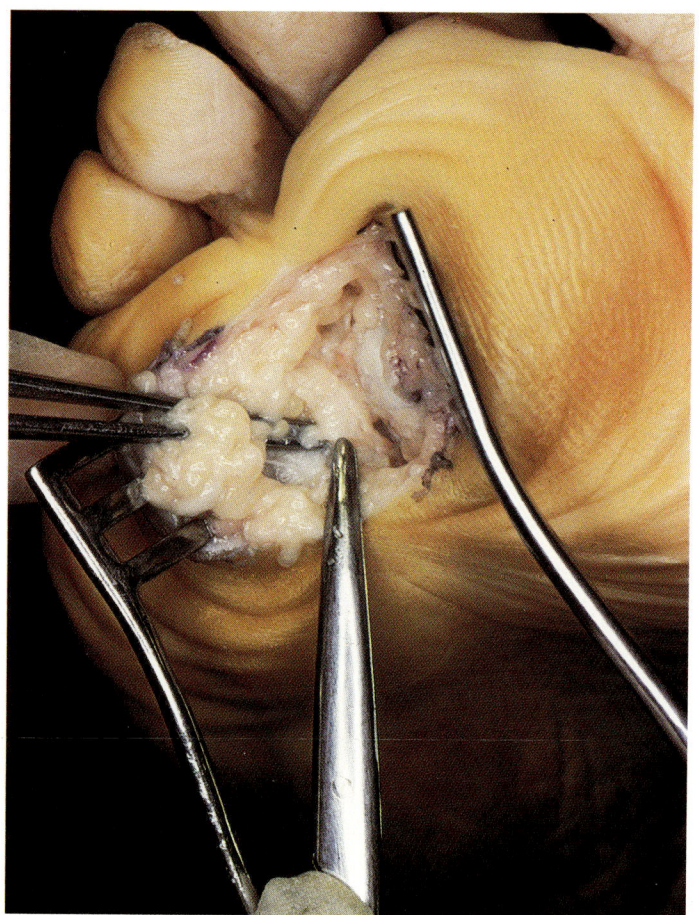

88 The nerve is identified by blunt dissection where it divides into the digital nerves to the adjacent toes. The nerve may lie quite deeply between the metatarsal heads and must be identified clearly. This part of the operation can be quite difficult and time-consuming.

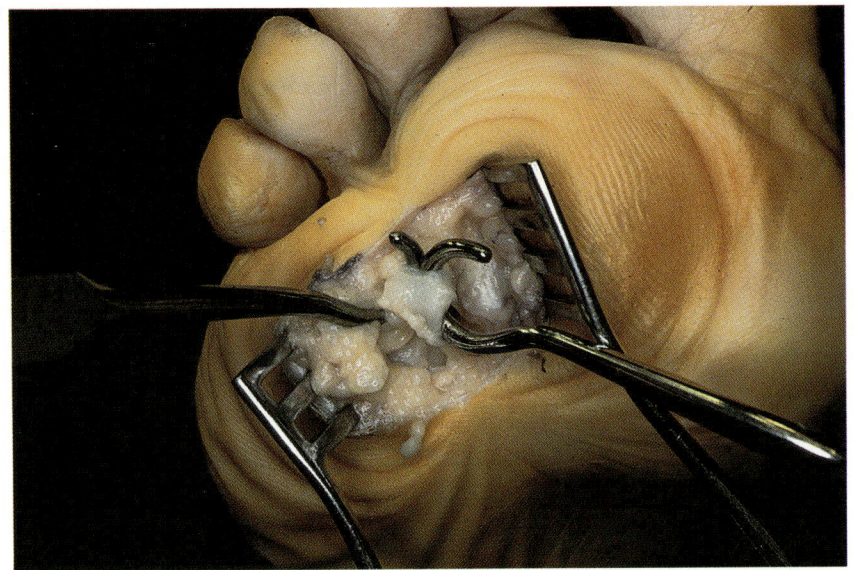

89 The digital nerves are drawn into the wound with hooks. The digital arteries lie deep to the nerves and are not at risk if the nerves are properly identified.

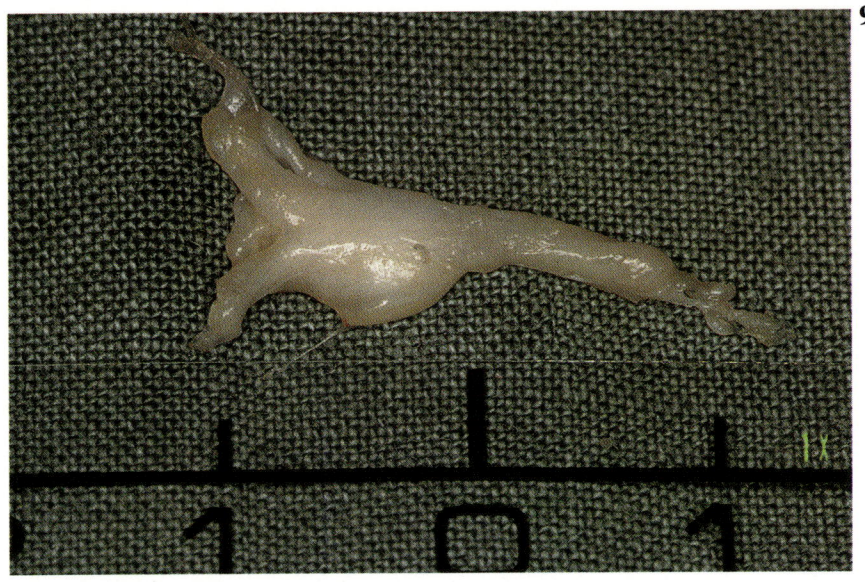

90 The 'neuroma'. A knife is used to divide the two digital nerves and traction will draw the plantar nerve into view. The plantar nerve should be divided at least 1 cm proximal to the swelling and the stump allowed to retract. Skin only is closed with 3–0 nylon sutures.

Postoperative management

A light wool and crepe dressing is applied. Heel walking is allowed but the foot should be kept elevated as much as possible. Normal footwear may be worn when the stitches are removed 14 days after operation.

Complications

Specific complications are infrequent. If an insufficient length of the plantar nerve is removed proximal to the neuroma, the stump of the nerve may become adherent to the transverse metatarsal ligament and cause recurrent symptoms.

Ablation of the nail

This operation (Zadik's procedure) is indicated for the treatment of onychogryphosis or recurrent ingrowing toenails. It is based on the fact that only the proximal part of the nailbed is responsible for the growth of the nail; resection of the nailbed from the convex border of the lunula to the base of the nailfold will prevent further growth. If an ingrowing toenail is infected, the nail should first be avulsed and Zadik's procedure deferred for two weeks.

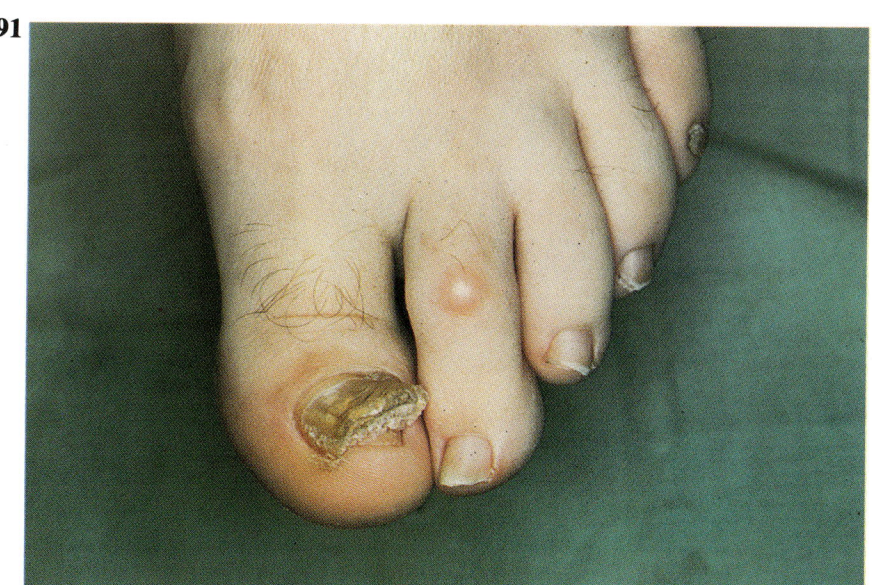

91 Onychogryphosis. The thickened, curved great toenail had been trimmed back with some difficulty, but wearing normal shoes was still uncomfortable.

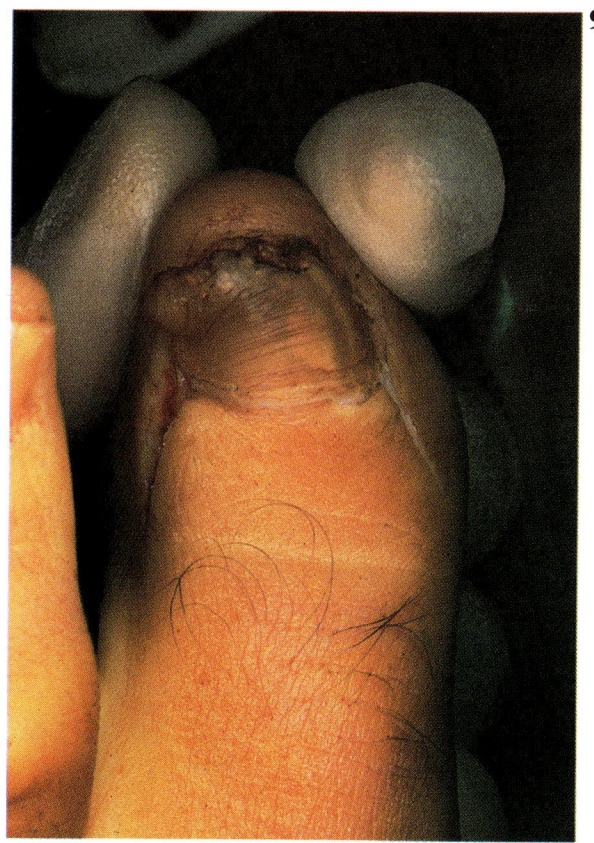

92 A 1 cm incision is made at each side of the base of the toenail.

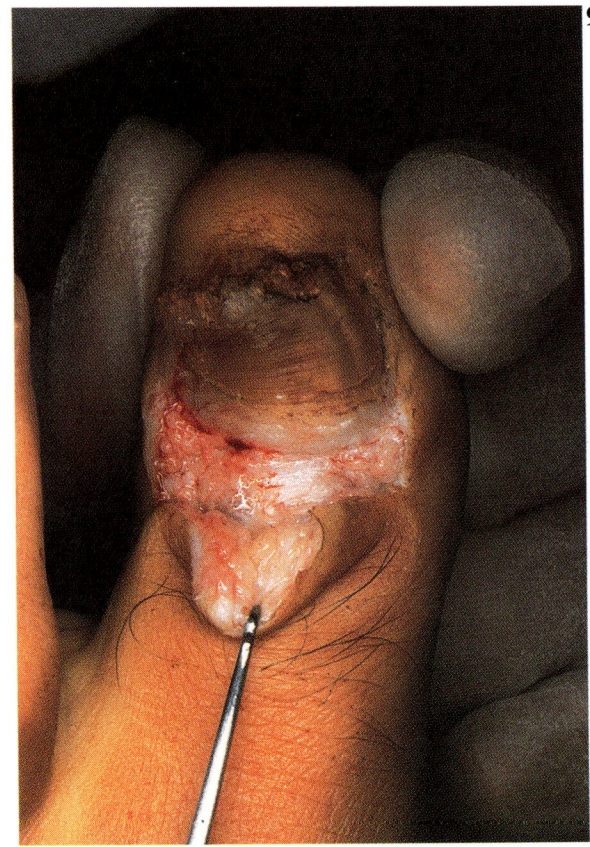

93 The flap is dissected back exposing the proximal border of the nail.

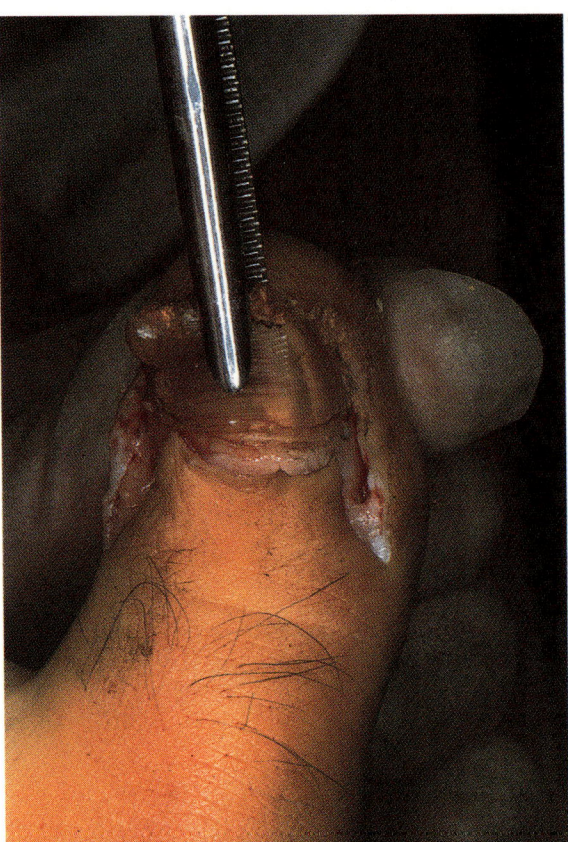

94 The nail is avulsed with stout forceps.

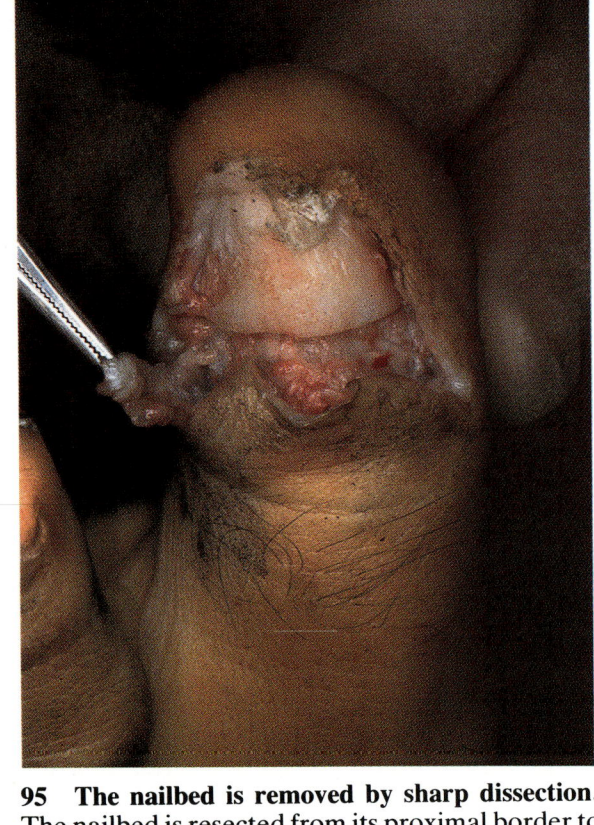

95 The nailbed is removed by sharp dissection. The nailbed is resected from its proximal border to just distal to the lunula (the white crescent seen under the normal nail), particular attention being paid to the proximal lateral recesses. The nailbed is removed down to the bone distally; proximally the dissection must be kept superficial to the extensor tendon. It is very easy to divide this and enter the interphalangeal joint if great care is not exercised.

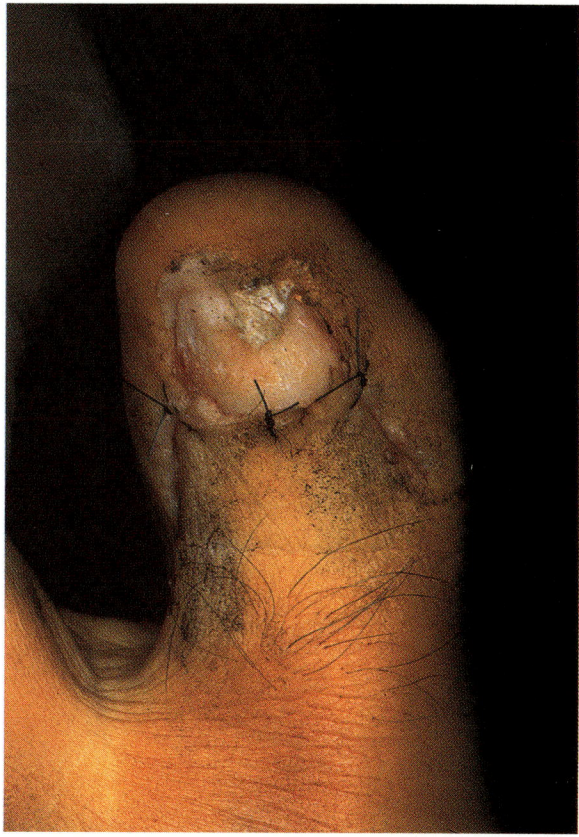

96 The skin flap is advanced to cover the area from which the nailbed has been resected. Tension should be avoided. The flap is held in place with a few 3–0 nylon sutures. The digital nerves are blocked with bupivacaine.

Postoperative management

A non-adherent dry dressing is applied. The foot is kept elevated as much as possible, although heel walking is permitted. Sutures are removed 8 days after operation; a protective dry dressing may be necessary for a few days longer.

Complications

Superficial infection is not uncommon; antibiotic treatment may be necessary if there are signs of cellulitis.

If the interphalangeal joint is inadvertently opened, it should be closed with fine absorbable sutures.

Partial regrowth of the nail will occur if the resection has been inadequate.

References

Cockin, J. (1968) 'Butler's operation for an overriding toe'.
Journal of Bone and Joint Surgery, **50B:**78–81.

Dinley, J. and Dickson, R.A. (1976) 'The control of pain after Keller's operation by the instillation of local anaesthetic before closure'.
Journal of Bone and Joint Surgery, **58B:**356–358.

Edmonson, A.S. and Crenshaw, A.H. (1980) *Campbell's Operative Orthopaedics,* (6th Ed).
C.V. Mosby Company, St Louis, Missouri.

Helal, B. (1975) 'Metatarsal osteotomy for metatarsalgia'.
Journal of Bone and Joint Surgery, **57B:**187–192.

Klenerman, L. (1982) *The Foot and Its Disorders,* (2nd Ed).
Blackwell Scientific Publications, Oxford.

Mitchell, C.L., Fleming, J.L., Allen, R., Glenney, C. and Sandford, G.A. (1958) 'Osteotomy-bunionectomy for hallux valgus'.
Journal of Bone and Joint Surgery, **40A:**41–59.

Nissen, K.I. (1948) 'Plantar digital neuritis: Morton's metatarsalgia'.
Journal of Bone and Joint Surgery, **30B:**84–94.

Thomas, F.B. (1963) 'Keller's arthroplasty modified'.
Journal of Bone and Joint Surgery, **44B:**356–365.

Zadik, F.R. (1950) 'Obliteration of the nailbed of the great toe without shortening of the terminal phalanx'.
Journal of Bone and Joint Surgery, **32B:**66–67.

Index

All figures refer to page numbers

A

Ablation of the nail 59
– complications of 61
– postoperative management of 61
Anaesthesia 9
Analgesia 12
Arthrodesis
– of first metatarsophalangeal joint 13
– complications of 23, 29
– postoperative management of 23, 29
– of interphalangeal joints 24

B

Bupivacaine 12
Butler's operation 51
– complications of 55
– postoperative management of 55

C

Callosity 24, 30, 35
Collodion 29

D

Dexon 29, 40, 46, 49
Dorsiflexion 14
Draping 10, 11

E

Esmarch bandage 9
'Exostosis' 35
Extensor hallucic longus tendon 15, 40

F

Fibrous union 29

H

Haematoma 23
Hallux rigidus 13
Hallux valgus 35, 42
Hammer toe 24
Helal osteotomy 30

I

Infection 23, 61
Ingrowing toenail 91

K

Keller's arthroplasty 35
– complications of 41
– postoperative management of 41
Kirschner wires 7, 20, 27, 40

L

Lunula 60

M

Mallet toe 24
Malposition 23
Metatarsalgia 30, 50
Mitchell's osteotomy 42
– complications of 50
– postoperative management of 50
Morton's neuroma 56

N

Nailbed 59
Non-union 23

O

Onychogryphosis 91
Osteoarthrosis 13
Osteophyte 13
Osteotomy
– of first metatarsal bone 42
– of metatarsal bones 30
– – complications of 34
– – postoperative management of 34
Over-riding fifth toe 51
Over-riding second toe 35

P

Plantar digital neuroma 51
Plaster 23, 34, 56
Powered burr 18
Powered saw 42, 47

R

References 62

S

Skin preparation 9
Stiffness of joints 34
Swelling 23

T

Tourniquet 9

V

Vicryl 29, 40, 46, 49

Z

Zadik's procedure 59